Acta Neurochirurgica
Supplement

Editor: H.-J. Steiger

Stereotactic and Functional Neurosurgery

Edited by
Guido Nikkhah and Marcus Pinsker

Acta Neurochirurgica
Supplement 117

Springer

Guido Nikkhah
and
Marcus Pinsker
Department of Neurosurgery
Division of Stereotactic and Functional
University Medical Center Freiburg
Freiburg, Germany

SpringerWienNewYork is part of Springer Science+Business Media
springer.at

Typesetting: SPI, Pondichery, India
Printed on acid-free and chlorine-free bleached paper

Library of Congress Control Number: 2013938369

With 27 (partly coloured) Figures

Additional material to this book can be downloaded from http://extras.springer.com

ISSN 0065-1419
ISBN 978-3-7091-1481-0   ISBN 978-3-7091-1482-7 (eBook)
DOI 10.1007/978-3-7091-1482-7
Springer Wien Heidelberg New York Dordrecht London

Foreword

More than 60 years ago, Traugott Riechert, Max Wolff, and Fritz Mundinger inaugurated a new targeting device for intracerebral interventions which later became world- famous as the *Riechert–Mundinger stereotactic system*. This was the basis for an important development in the history of stereotactic and functional neurosurgery. One of the first milestone operations with this system was performed on November 14, 1952. During this day, the Freiburg team performed for the first time in the history of medicine a neurosurgical operation by stereotactic means to lesion a deeply seated nucleus of the basal ganglia. It was Fritz Mundinger who performed this surgery in the presence of Wolf Hassler, Traugott Riechert, and R. von Baumgarten on a 38-year-old man who suffered from Parkinson's disease with severe tremor. It was the first thalamotomy, and marks an important date in the history of functional neurosurgery for movement disorders.

From this time on, stereotactic and functional neurosurgery have evolved into a fascinating and interdisciplinary endeavour that combines modern neurosurgery, neurobiology, and neuroimaging with innovative diagnostic and treatment strategies. During the International Congress on the occasion of the 60th Anniversary of Stereotactic and Functional Neurosurgery in Freiburg, we celebrated these pioneering and outstanding achievements with a series of lectures that were given by the different generations of neurosurgeons, including the fathers of modern stereotaxy, among them Philipp Gildenberg and Ronald Tasker. During the 3 days of the Congress from December 1 to December 3, 2011, a great international audience were able to witness the ground-breaking and exciting journey that pioneers in stereotactic and functional neurosurgery have undertaken until today to conquer the challenges imposed by the diseases of the human nervous system, such as pain, movement disorders, brain tumors, and psychiatric diseases.

Following this 60th Anniversary Meeting of Stereotactic Neurosurgery in Freiburg, a number of authors were invited to contribute to this dedicated volume of *Acta Neurochirurgica*. I am very happy that 16 authors have compiled their scientific and clinical experience in stereotactic and functional neurosurgery, in movement disorders, and in brain tumors. The scientific contributions present a wide range from the beginnings of human stereotactic neurosurgery to the most modern molecular and restorative strategies to treat diseases of the human nervous system. They also clearly exemplify that the discipline of stereotactic and functional neurosurgery is still a young and dynamic discipline, with alternative and sometimes competing neurosurgical and functional neurosurgical strategies that are still under further evaluation. They also document that operative lesioning techniques such as thalamotomies have been succeeded by novel neuromodulation techniques such as deep brain stimulation in the great majority of clinical cases. However, under some circumstances, the older techniques have still their place in modern functional neurosurgery.

Anyone who is further interested in the specific circumstances of the development of the Department of Stereotactic and Functional Neurosurgery in Freiburg over the 60 years is referred to the book that was published under the title "Journeys to the center of the brain" by Guido Nikkhah in collaboration with Julia Bidder and Walter Birg.

It is my special privilege to thank all the authors and co-authors of this volume for their valuable scientific contribution. I want to express my sincere gratitude to my co-workers Marcus Pinsker, Thomas Reithmeier, Michael Trippel, and Thomas Prokop for their invaluable help in the review of the manuscripts as well as in the editorial work. A big thank you belongs to Manuela Fellmann who supported me during the preparation of this dedicated volume. Many thanks belong to the European Society for Stereotactic and Functional Neurosurgery, the staff members of Acta Neurochirurgica, especially the editor Hans-Jakob Steiger, all of whom were very helpful and supportive in the finalization of this project. Last, but not least, I am especially thankful to the Sponsors of the Anniversary Meeting for their invaluable financial contribution, and among them especially to the Medtronic company which, in addition, financially supported the publication of this dedicated volume.

I want to dedicate this supplement volume to Fritz Mundinger who died at the age of 87 on May 23, 2012. His clinical and scientific contributions laid an important ground in my own career in stereotactic and functional neurosurgery. I had the privilege to learn from his sharp and brilliant mind and clinical skills over many years, and I truly enjoyed the intense personal discussions I had with him over all these years, even until a few weeks before he died. His contributions to stereotactic and functional neurosurgery will remain a major hallmark for many generations of young neurosurgeons to come, and the present volume of *Acta Neurochirurgica* is a fine example of his unique inheritance. May it direct our attention to the right "targets" during the further progress of this exciting and fascinating journey towards the human brain and its best treatments for our patients.

Freiburg, July 17th, 2012 Guido Nikkhah

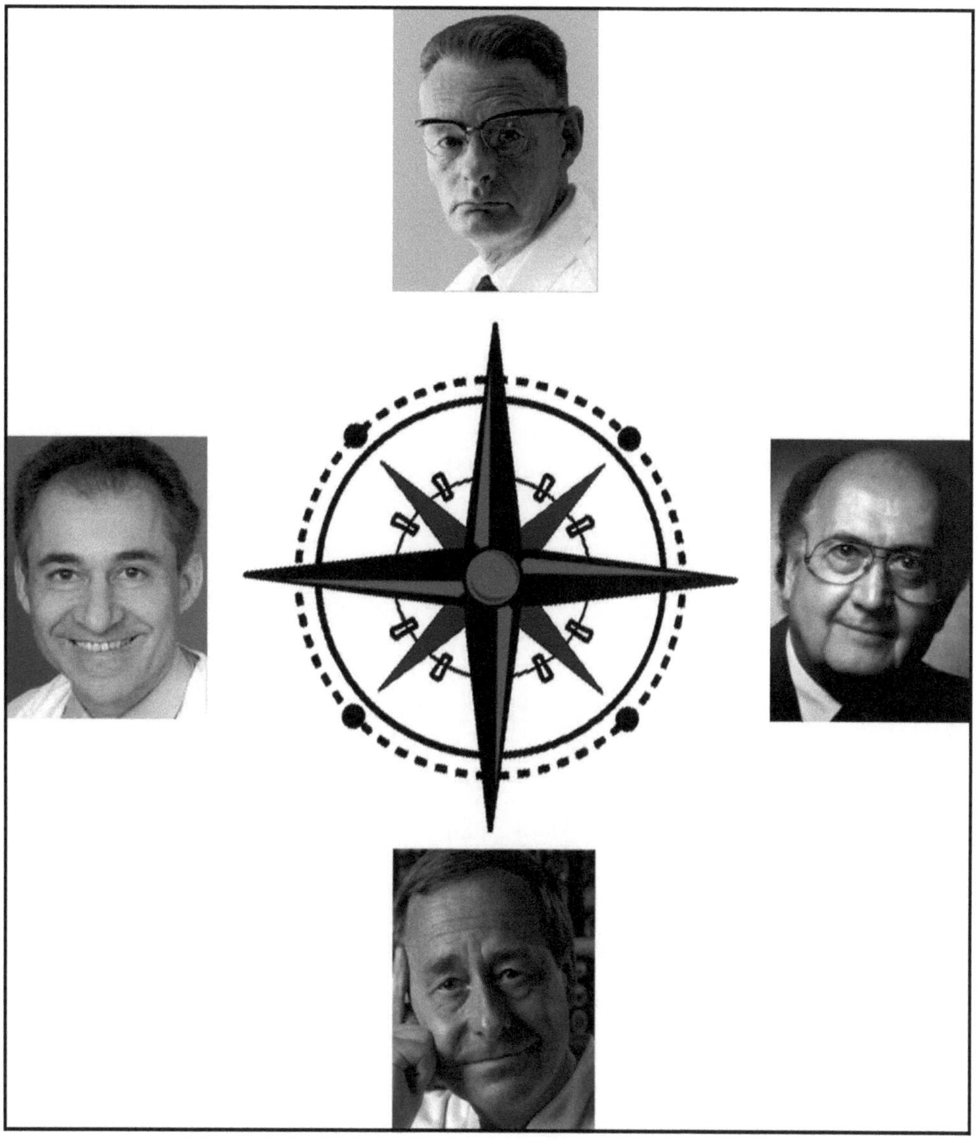

Contents

The Birth of Human Stereotactic Surgery

Philip L. Gildenberg

Abstract Stereotactic surgery began with the Horsley–Clarke apparatus which has been used in animal research since 1908. In 1947, Spiegel and Wycis introduced stereotactic surgery in human patients. Their initial choice of target involved the extrapyramidal system, which Russell Meyers had recently performed with craniotomy and manual lesions that might alleviate symptoms of movement disorders, albeit with significant morbidity and mortality, a problem not seen with stereotactic surgery.

Keywords Cartesian coordinates • Extrapyramidal system • Horsley and Clarke stereotaxic apparatus (animal research) • Huntington's chorea • International Society for Research in Stereoencephalotomy • Pallidotomy • Pneumoencephalographic landmarks • Psychosurgery • Russell Meyers • Spiegel and Wycis stereotactic apparatus (human patients) • Stereotaxic surgery • World Society for Stereotactic and Functional Neurosurgery

Animal stereotactic surgery pre-dated human stereotactic surgery by almost 40 years. Why did it take so long to apply this accurate minimally invasive technique to human patients? To find the logical explanation, it is necessary to look at the state of several arts that came together at just the right time — advances in knowledge of physiology of the nervous system, a desire to perform a discredited neurosurgical procedure with accuracy and better patient selection, and advances in radiology that made it possible to identify landmarks in the brain from which accurate target placement could be defined.

The birth of animal stereotactic surgery occurred in 1908, when Horsley and Clarke [1] reported on a device for inserting a needle or electrode accurately into a desired structure in the monkey brain. The animal's head was secured by two ear plugs and by two tabs that held the inferior orbital rims; thus, the ear plugs assured accurate alignment with the midline. The orbital tabs held the head in a reproducibly accurate position. The three planes which formed the Cartesian planes were the midplane, the basal or horizontal plane that passed through the ear plugs and the orbital tabs, and the zero coronal plane that formed right angles to the other two planes and passed through the ear plugs. In the material and methods section of the landmark article, the Horsley and Clarke not only described the stereotactic apparatus but a method to make a stereotactic atlas. The description of forming a reproducible electrolytic lesion in itself was a significant contribution. To conclude on a high note, there was a study of the physiology of the cerebellum of the monkey.

Since localization of the target was dependent on the configuration of structures in the skull, which are consistent within each breed of experimental animals, accurate placement was almost assured. In addition, localization was verified by sectioning the brain when the animal was sacrificed, and data from unsatisfactory placement could be discarded.

It was fortunate that they did not use that type of device on human patients, since they recognized that the human skull is much too variable to assure an accurately placed target. An engineer, Mussen, did, however, design and produce a prototype according to the dimensions of the human head. Fortunately, he did not find a surgeon to use it clinically. The error would have been so great that it might have set back the development of stereotaxis even further.

What were some of the intellectual impediments to the development of human basal ganglia surgery between 1908 and 1940? In 1940, it was thought that surgery on the basal ganglia would cause permanent impairment of consciousness. This was based on assertion by Dandy [2], on observation of two patients, that occlusion of the left anterior cerebral artery and the distribution of the resultant cerebral damage caused permanent loss of consciousness (although his description is

P.L. Gildenberg, MD, PhD
Restoration Robotics, Inc., Houston Stereotactic Concepts, Inc., 3776 Darcus Street, Houston, TX 77005, USA
e-mail: hscp@sbcglobal.net

G. Nikkhah and M. Pinsker (eds.), *Stereotactic and Functional Neurosurgery*, Acta Neurochirurgica Supplement, Vol. 117,
DOI 10.1007/978-3-7091-1482-7_1, © Springer-Verlag Wien 2013

more like the locked-in state). Consequently, Dandy advocated against basal ganglia surgery or any surgery damaging to the left hemisphere near the corpus callosum [3], since he believed that surgery to the left anterior lobe posterior to the corpus callosum would result in permanent unconsciousness. This truism advocated against basal ganglia surgery, and persisted throughout most of the 1940s.

Bucy [4, 5], a vocal early pioneer in movement disorder surgery, insisted throughout that it was necessary to interrupt the primary motor cortex and its descending tracts to alleviate tremor. The recognized side-effects to those tracts occurred, so the rationale indicated that it was worth trading hemiplegia, spasticity, and contractures for tremor. In the absence of other therapy, either surgical or pharmacological, this was apparently considered a good trade-off. Bucy [6] continued to advocate pyramidal ablation even after successful stereotactic surgery was introduced.

From the practical standpoint, we must note that the majority of patients with movement disorders that were referred to surgeons had Parkinson's disease or sometimes Huntingdon's chorea. There were no effective pharmacological agents, there were a huge number of Parkinsonian patients, many of whom had a history of encephalitis during the epidemics 20 years previously, and tremor was the one sign that could be demonstrated most readily in order to recognize improvement.

Thus, in 1940, we have two giants in the field advocating against the very basal ganglia surgery that later became the basis for stereotactic surgery for movement disorders.

What happened between 1940 and 1947 to change significantly the surgical approach to movement disorders?

The reason that I emphasize 1940 as the comparison date is that we have an excellent snap-shot of knowledge of the basal ganglia at precisely that time. A meeting chaired by Tracy Putnam on "The Diseases of Basal Ganglia" was held in New York under the auspices of the Association for Research in Nervous and Mental Disease on December 20 and 21, 1940. The original proceedings appeared in 1942, but the entire transcripts were re-published by Hafner Publishing Company in New York in 1966, including the discussion of most papers that was heard at the 1940 meeting [7].

The speakers at the 1940 meeting were the giants in their respective fields, whose contributions constituted the state of the art. Speakers included Lewy, Papez, the Ransons, Mettler, Fulton, Merritt, Klemme, and Russell Meyers, (who was not well known at that time), with closing remarks by Putnam. Spiegel was not listed to be in attendance and Wycis was too junior to be invited, although it is certain that they were very aware of the knowledge that was exchanged.

The meeting began with an erudite review of the history of the basal ganglia by Lewy [8], citing its first description by Thomas Willis in 1664, which included a drawing of the sheep basal ganglia by Christopher Wren, the great seventeenth century English architect. That article first used the terms corpus striatum, lentiform bodies and thalamus.

Lewy quoted that the Willis manuscript opined that "the corpus striatum represents an exchange between brain stem and cortex". Lewy quoted Edinger as saying almost 250 years later that "We lack any knowledge of the function of the corpus striatum or of the symptoms following its stimulation or destruction. Lewy also cited his own 1912 manuscript reported that "after one hundred years of laborious preliminary studies the 'Gestalt' of the basal ganglia, their function and diseases became suddenly visible around the year 1912" [9], 4 years after the introduction of the Horsley–Clarke apparatus, but there was still disagreement about the relationship of the basal ganglia as to function and the relationship to motor disorders [8].

Foerster reiterated at the 1940 meeting that the corpus striatum is a center for the integration of elemental movement patterns into hierarchies of automatic associated acts [10].

A few years before the 1940 Meeting, in 1937, Magoun et al. [11] suggested that emotional expression, at least in part, is subtended by the basal ganglia, but gave little emphasis to motor control, as demonstrated by Meyers [12] at the 1940 meeting.

We cannot leave the history of surgical treatment for movement disorders prior to 1940 without acknowledging those procedures that did not involve the basal ganglia, or even the brain. To present a few examples, Foerster suggested posterior rhizotomy for treatment of tremor [13]. Royle reported on sympathectomy as a treatment for movement disorders in 1924 [14]. Puusepp advocated dorsal column section for a variety of movement disorders [15]. Almost any part of the nervous system was attacked in futile attempts to alleviate motor disorders. Even today, we have only little information about many of the motor disorders that do not have an animal model for research; it is common to attempt treatment with interruption or stimulation of a variety of targets, most of which involve the brain stem.

Let us return to the 1940 meeting. Bucy continued to endorse ablation of the motor cortex or pyramidal tract, trading hemiplegia, spasticity, dyspraxia, hyperreflexia, clonus, and spreading reflex synergies for alleviation of motor disorders, especially tremor of Parkinson's disease. He indicated that improvement in motor disease is not possible without involving ablation of the motor cortex or its related tracts [5].

No one considered challenging Dandy's admonition against surgery of the basal ganglia until Russell Meyers [16] spoke. As probably the most junior participant is the discussion, his presentation was scheduled just before the chairman Putnam's final paper, which included a concluding summary of the meeting [7].

Meyers was then an instructor in Neurophysiology and Neurology at the Long Island College of Medicine, as well as Assistant Neurosurgeon at several New York Hospitals, and he later became Professor of Neurosurgery at the University of Iowa Medical School.

During 1939 and 1940, Meyers [12, 16] performed the first successful extrapyramidal surgery for treatment of unilateral tremor of Parkinsonism. There were eight patients in all; each reported with a complete neurological history, but only one of the patients was treated with sufficient success to advocate the use of brain stem surgery. All patients were operated while awake, as was most common in the neurosurgery of those days. Since there no localizing devices, the plan was to use the ventricular anatomy to visualize what was probably the head of the caudate nucleus. A right frontal craniotomy was performed and the lateral ventricle entered, except in one patient where there was difficulty finding the ventricle with a brain cannula. In the second patient, the improvement was encouraging, but only temporary, so three craniotomies over 4 months were performed with only modest improvement. Other targets were used in the next three patients, with only slight improvement.

In all patients, an attempt was made to extirpate the head or part of the head of the caudate nucleus, but in several, there was also damage to the anterior limb of the internal capsule. The final two patients appeared also to have section of the ansa lenticularis with very good to excellent results, but the seventh patient developed a craniotomy wound infection which proved fatal on the eighth postoperative day.

The eighth patient reported at that meeting was operated on December 3, 1940, just 3 weeks before the meeting. She had section of the ansa lenticularis and some of the lenticular funiculus, so probably the adjacent globus pallidus had also been injured. She was described as having an "excellent result" with no qualifications. It is interesting to note that the first targeted procedure employed by Spiegel and Wycis 7 years later was not a pallidotomy, but a pallido-ansotomy, similar to the lesion made by Meyers' open surgery.

Meyers continued to perform the transventricular approach to the caudate and globus pallidus, and reported 58 patients in proceedings of a subsequent meeting [17]. By that time, stereotactic surgery had been demonstrated, and Meyers opined that the 12 % risk of open surgery was too great to be justified.

What was demonstrated by Meyers' case reports? Success could be achieved without encroaching on the primary motor fibers — *Bucy was wrong*. The patients had no impairment of consciousness after resecting or lesioning a structure within the brain stem — *Dandy was wrong*. The door was opened to the development of human stereotactic surgery.

Another seemingly unrelated milestone occurred between 1940 and 1947. Intraoperative radiology became practical. It was possible to take an X-ray and have the developed film returned to the OR in as little as 10 min. The definition was good enough to identify an air-filled third ventricle, so intracerebral landmarks could be used.

The field of animal stereotaxic surgery as a means of studying neurophysiology advanced steadily from the time of Horsley and Clarke's [1] introduction of the method, but human stereotaxis was not introduced for 39 years afterward. The significant difference between animal and human stereotactic surgery concerned the way landmarks were localized in three-dimensional Cartesian space. The animal headholder not only secured the animal's head in proper alignment, but provided the references to measure the coordinates of the target. Human stereotactic surgery relied on landmarks within the brain, such as the mid-plane, and the anterior and posterior commissures to establish a frame of reference. This distinction was great enough that Spiegel and Wycis originally called this new technique "stereoencephalotomy", that is, using the anatomy of the encephalon to establish the basic coordinates.

The stage was set to introduce human stereotactic surgery.

The first Spiegel–Wycis apparatus was essentially a Horsley–Clarke apparatus mounted on a head ring that was secured to the patient's head by an individually made plaster cap with a hole in the middle. The article appeared in *Science* [18], along with two views of the apparatus.

The original motivation to develop human stereotactic surgery was to perform more refined pre-frontal lobotomy for psychiatric disease, for instance by making a controlled lesion in the dorsomedial nucleus of the thalamus. However, by the time that human stereotaxis appeared, pre-frontal lobotomy had fallen out of favor.

The first procedure was pallido-ansotomy for Huntington's chorea, with good results and no neurological complications. During the first 4 years the mortality rate was less than 1 %, which has fallen to less than 0.5 % thereafter, during which time basal ganglia surgery became the accepted procedure for motor disorders.

Often overlooked is the last paragraph of the 1947 paper in *Science* [18].

"This apparatus is being used for psychosurgery... Lesions have been placed in the region of the medial nucleus of the thalamus (medial thalamotomy)... Further applications of the stereotaxic technique are under study, e.g., interruption of the spinothalamic tract in certain types of pain or phantom limb; production of pallidal lesions in involuntary movements; electrocoagulation of the Gasserian ganglion in trigeminal neuralgia; and withdrawal of fluid from pathological cavities, cystic tumors." Spiegel was especially secretive about ongoing projects, so I am certain that all of those procedures had been done prior to that first publication [18].

One might ask why the first patient had Huntington's chorea rather than Parkinson's disease. Kennard and Fulton had observed paucity of movements in primates after pallidal lesions [19] and Spiegel and Wycis were concerned that pallidotomy might make parkinsonian bradykinesia worse.

It was not until Hassler and Riechert in 1951 demonstrated that a lesion in the ventrolateral thalamus near the site of the pallidofugal fibers could safely and effectively manage Parkinson's disease that thalamotomy was accepted as a target for Parkinson's disease and other movement [20–22].

There were several basal ganglia targets developed during the first few years. Pallidotomy, actually pallidotomy–ansotomy, became the most common target for Parkinson's disease [23, 24]. In 1952 Spiegel and Wycis compared mesencephalotomy, thalamotomy and pallidotomy [25]. In 1963 they reported making a lesion in Forel's field, which they named campotomy, as their favored target for Parkinson's disease [26].

The status of human stereotactic surgery was reviewed in 1952 in a book, *Stereoencephalotomy, Part I*, by Spiegel and Wycis, which included the first human stereotactic atlas [27]. A decade later they wrote *Stereoencephalotomy, Part II* [28], which documented some of the tremendous progress made during the first decade of human stereotactic surgery, progress that is occurring at an ever more rapid rate.

So what happened between 1940 and 1947? Basic anatomy and some physiology of the basal ganglia had advanced. Russell Meyers proved that basal ganglia surgery could be done without impairing consciousness and could be used as a treatment for Parkinson's disease. Intraoperative X-ray was introduced.

The stage was set for human stereotactic surgery to be born.

Conflict of Interest We declare that we have no conflict of interest.

References

1. Horsley V, Clarke RH (1908) The structure and functions of the cerebellum examined by a new method. Brain 31:45–124
2. Dandy WE (1966) The brain. W.F. Prior Company, Hagerstown
3. Meyers R (1951) Dandy's striatal theory of the "center of consciousness"; surgical evidence and logical analysis indicating its improbability. AMA Arch Neurol Psychiatry 65:659–671
4. Bucy PC, Case TJ (1939) Tremor. Physiologic mechanism and abolition by surgical means. Arch Neurol Psychiatry 41:721–746
5. Bucy PC (1966) Cortical extirpation in the treatment of involuntary movements. In: Putnam TJ (ed) The diseases of the basal ganglia. Hafner Publishing Co., New York, pp 551–595
6. Bucy PC (1970) The surgical treatment of abnormal involuntary movements. J Neurosurg Nurs 2:31–39
7. Putnam TJ (ed) (1966) The diseases of the basal ganglia. Hafner Publishing Co., New York
8. Lewy FH (1966) Historical introduction: the basal ganglia and their diseases. In: Putnam TJ (ed) The diseases of the basal ganglia. Hafner Publishing Co., New York, pp 1–20
9. Lewy FH (1912) Die pathologischen Anatomie der Paralysis agitans. Lewandowskys Handb 3:920
10. Foerster O (1921) Zur Anayse und Pathophysiologie der striären Bewegungsstörungen. Ztschr Neurol Psychiatr 73:1
11. Magoun HW, Atlas D, Ingersoll EH, Ranson SW (1937) Associated facial, vocal and respiratory components of emotional expression: an experimental study. J Neurol Psychopathol 17:241
12. Meyers R (1966) The modification of alternating tremors, rigidity and festination by surgery of the basal ganglia. In: Putnam TJ (ed) The diseases of the basal ganglia. Hafner Publishing Co., New York, pp 602–665
13. Foerster O (1913) On the indications and results of the excision of posterior spinal nerve roots in men. Surg Gynecol Obstet 16:463–475
14. Royle ND (1924) A new operative procedure in the treatment of spastic paralysis and its experimental basis. Med J Aust 1:77–86
15. Puusepp L (1930) Cordotomia posterior lateralis (fasc. Burdachi) on account of trembling and hypertonia of the muscles of the hand. Folia Neuropath Estomiona 10:62
16. Meyers R (1940) Surgical procedure for postencephalitic tremor, with notes on the physiology of premotor fibers. Arch Neurol Psychiatry 44:455–459
17. Meyers R (1958) Historical background and personal experiences in the surgical relief of hyperkinesia and hypertonus. In: Fields W (ed) Pathogenesis and treatment of Parkinsonism. Chas C. Thomas, Springfield, pp 229–270
18. Spiegel EA, Wycis HT, Marks M, Lee AS (1947) Stereotaxic apparatus for operations on the human brain. Science 106:349–350
19. Kennard MA, Fulton JF (1966) Corticostriatal interrelations in monkey and chimpanzee. In: Putnam TJ (ed) The diseases of the basal ganglia. Hafner Publishing Co., New York, pp 228–245
20. Hassler R, Riechert T (1954) Indikationen und Lokalisationsmethode der gezielten Hirnoperationen. Nervenarzt 25:441–447
21. Hassler R, Riechert T (1955) A special method of stereotactic brain operation. Proc R Soc Med 48:469–470
22. Hassler R, Hess WR (1954) Experimentelle und anatomische Befunde über die Drehbewegungen und die nervösen Apparate. Arch Psychiatr Nervenkr 192:488–526
23. Spiegel EA, Wycis HT (1950) Pallido-thalamotomy in chorea. Arch Neurol Psychiatry 64:495–496
24. Spiegel EA, Wycis HT (1952) Thalamotomy and pallidotomy for treatment of choreic movements. Acta Neurochir [Wien] 2: 417–422
25. Spiegel EA, Wycis HT, Freed H (1952) Stereoencephalotomy in thalamotomy and related procedures. J Am Med Assoc 148: 446–451
26. Spiegel EA, Wycis HT, Szekely EG, Baird HW III, Adams J, Flanagan M (1962) Campotomy. Trans Am Neurol Assoc 87:240–242
27. Spiegel EA, Wycis HT (1952) Stereoencephalotomy, part I. Grune & Stratton, New York
28. Spiegel EA, Wycis HT (1962) Sterencephalotomy, part II. Grune & Stratton, New York

Functional Neurosurgery in Parkinson's Disease: A Long Journey from Destruction Over Modulation Towards Restoration

Guido Nikkhah, Gustavo Adolpho Carvalho, and Marcus Pinsker

Abstract Neurosurgical treatment of Parkinson's disease (PD) has re-gained considerable attention over the last two decades due to a better understanding of the pathophysiology of the basal ganglia, the long-term complications of medical treatment, and advances in neuroimaging and neurosurgical techniques. The introduction of deep brain stimulation (DBS) has created new perspectives for the surgical management of PD patients, due to the low morbidity, reversibility and improvement of both motor function and quality of life as compared to the lesioning techniques. We present an overview of basic principles, history, indications, and results of current neurosurgical techniques available in PD.

Keywords Parkinson's disease • Ablative techniques • Deep brain stimulation

G. Nikkhah, MD, PhD (✉)
Division of Stereotactic and Functional Neurosurgery,
Department of General Neurosurgery,
Neurosurgical Clinic, University Medical Center Freiburg,
Breisacher Straße 64, Freiburg D-79106, Germany

Neurosurgical Clinic,
University Hospital Erlangen,
Schwabachanlage 6, Erlangen D-91054, Germany
e-mail: guido.nikkhah@uk-erlangen.de

G.A. Carvalho
Department of Neurosurgery, Hospital Adventista Silvestre,
Rio de Janeiro Brazil, Rua Bambina 56 sala 105,
Botafogo, Rio de Janeiro, Brazil
e-mail: gustavoadolpho@neurocirurgioes.com.br

M. Pinsker, MD
Division of Stereotactic and Functional Neurosurgery,
Department of General Neurosurgery,
Neurosurgical Clinic, University Medical Center Freiburg,
Breisacher Straße 64, Freiburg D-79106, Germany

Klinik für Neurochirurgie, HELIOS Klinikum Berlin-Buch,
Schwanebecker Chaussee 50, Berlin DE-13125, Germany

Introduction

Parkinson's disease (PD) was first described as a clinical entity by James Parkinson in 1817, based principally on the observed patient's symptoms: tremor, flexed posture, movement impairment, and the time progression of the disease [18]. Idiopathic Parkinson's disease (IPD) is a clinical syndrome, which is based mainly on the following findings: akinesia or bradykinesia (expressed as the general poverty of movements), tremor (affecting 70–85 % of the patients, classically seen as piece-like or pill-rolling movements of the index and thumb with flexion–extension movements of the wrist), rigidity, postural instability, and autonomic disturbances. The incidence of Parkinson's disease shows a progressive and exponential age-related rise, with a prevalence of 2.2 % in the elderly population and an overall prevalence of 120–180 out of 100,000, with an annual incidence of 15–20 per 100,000 in Caucasian population. IPD is supposed to have a world prevalence of 10–405 out of 100,000 [1].

Pathophysiological changes in PD are based on the loss of dopaminergic cells in the substantia nigra pars compacta and a decrease of the normal nigrostriatal inhibition within the basal ganglia circuitry [14, 55, 57, 58]. Reduction of the inhibitory activity of the nigrostriatal pathway to the GABAergic striatal neurons leads to an overactivity of the striatal neurons, and consequently to a higher inhibition of the external segment of the globus pallidus (GPe) [7, 15]. Thus, there is an overactivity of the subthalamic nucleus (STN), due to the reduced activity of the inhibitory fibers from the GPe to the STN, resulting in an excessive glutamatergic input from the STN to the internal segment of the globus pallidus (GPi) and pars reticulata of the substantia nigra (SNr). Finally, increased activity of GPi and SNr leads to an excessive inhibition of the thalamus and then to a suppression of cortical activity via the thalamo-cortical projections, which is probably responsible,

G. Nikkhah and M. Pinsker (eds.), *Stereotactic and Functional Neurosurgery*, Acta Neurochirurgica Supplement, Vol. 117,
DOI 10.1007/978-3-7091-1482-7_2,

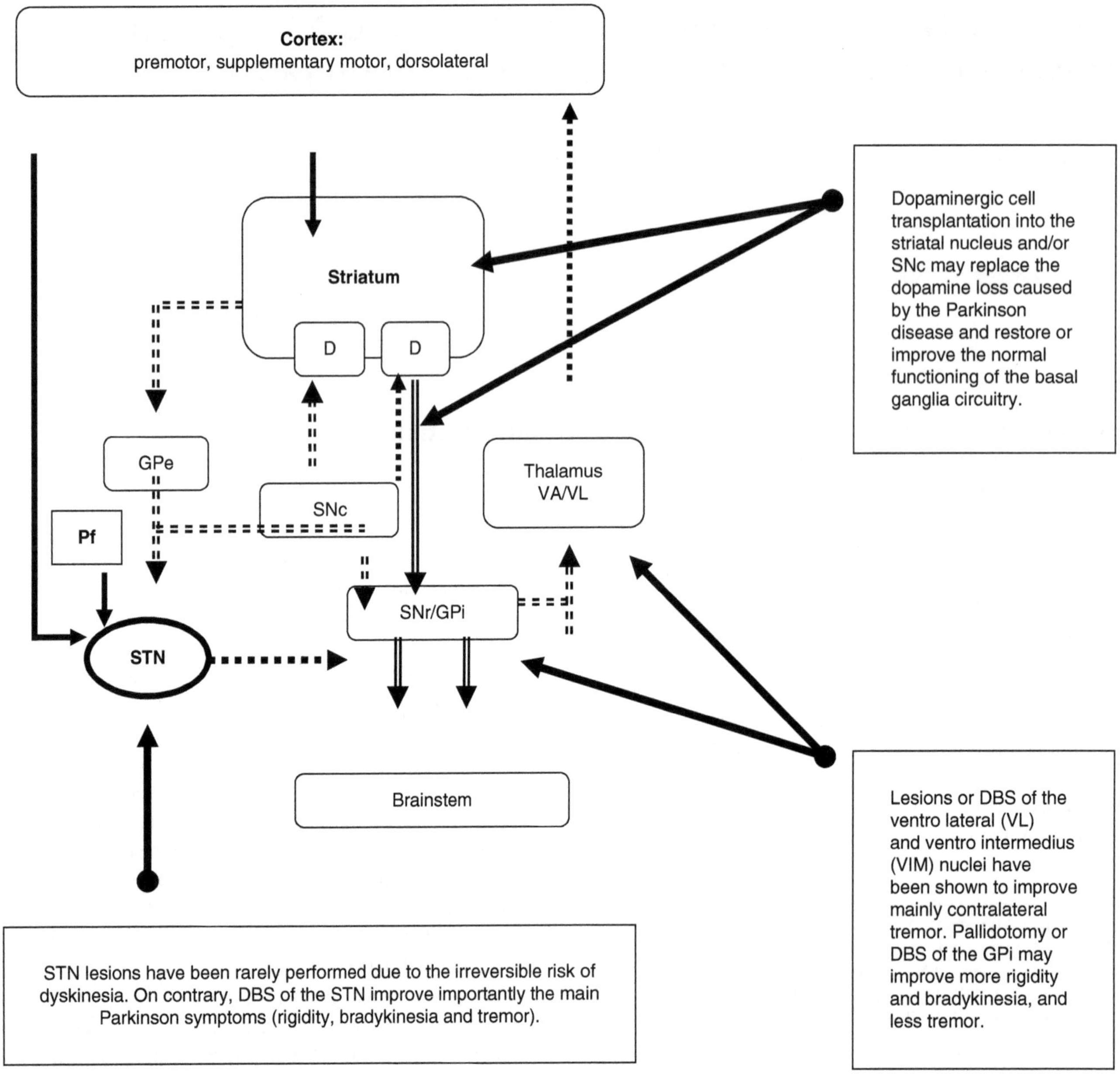

Fig. 1 Diagram showing the actual model of PD based on the loss of dopaminergic neurons in the SN pars compacta and the different targets for the surgical treatment in PD. *Interrupted arrows* represent the principally affected pathways in PD. Both Gpe and STN are hyper-activated due to the affecting of the inhibitory GABAergic pathways (– –).

at least in part, for the bradykinesia, tremor, and rigidity observed in parkinsonian patients.

Electrophysiological studies report no clear hypoactivity of the GPe in an animal model of Parkinson's disease, challenging the hypothesis that STN hyperactivity would be mainly due to the inhibition of the GPe and impairment of pallidal-subthalamic inhibitory fibers [10, 23, 25]. In fact, STN hyperactivity could be due also to other excitatory inputs, e.g., from the parafascicular nucleus and cortex [15].

Surgical Treatment of Parkinson's Disease

Surgical treatment of PD today can be divided into ablative procedures, neuromodulation (deep brain stimulation, DBS) and neural transplantation (Fig. 1). All require stereotactic techniques and equipment, which were developed at the beginning of the last century. The history of surgical interventions in PD dates back to 1908, when Horsley and Clarke introduced the first stereotactic apparatus on the basis of Cartesian coordinates. Since then it has been possible to place an electrode with high precision into any deep-located structure within the brain. The first stereotactic procedure in humans was performed by Spiegel and Wycis in 1947, using the so called "stereoencephalotome". This apparatus was used for placing a lesion in the region of the medial nucleus of the thalamus, to reduce emotional reactivity. That means that the first indication for stereotactic neurosurgery was a psychiatric indication. In the conclusion of their publication of the results of this procedure from the year 1947, the authors state further applications under study, e.g., interruption of the spinothalamic tract in pain, pallidal lesions in involuntary movements and electrocoagulation of the Gasserian ganglion in trigeminal neuralgia [62].

In different centers worldwide, several systems were developed almost in parallel, among them the first center-of arc-system by Lars Leksell in 1948, and in 1951 by Riechert and Wolff another center-of-arc-system, but this one including the first phantom to control the adjustments. Hassler and Riechert performed a ventro-lateral thalamotomy in 1951 in a patient with PD. Based on the results of microelectrode recordings, used intraoperatively during the lesioning for target localization, a detailed description of the nuclei was possible. Already in the 1960s it was observed that tremor could be suppressed very effectively with high-frequency stimulation in the ventral intermedius nucleus (VIM) of the thalamus, whereas the tremor was increased by low-frequency stimulation.

PD was, in the pre-levodopa era, a primarily surgically treated disease. The numbers of lesional procedures declined dramatically after the introduction of levodopa. Nevertheless, due to the long-term complications of levodopa therapy such as motor fluctuations and dyskinesias and in patients with intractable tremor, the need for further treatment options increased again.

The step to implanting neuromodulation systems required implantable hardware, which was not available before the 1980s. In 1987, Benabid et al. [6] performed the first DBS (unilateral) of the VIM, in combination with contralateral thalamotomy. The promising results led finally to DBS of the Gpi and, later, the STN in PD.

Parallel to the "symptomatic" therapy of lesioning or neuromodulation, a third technique is still under investigation. Since the basis of the disease is a loss of nigral cells in the substantia nigra, replacing these cells would (theoretically) solve the problem. Demonstrating the functional restoration with neural transplantation in the 1970s provided hope for neural repair. In two prospective U.S. studies with sham surgeries as controls during the 1990s there was no clinical benefit; moreover, some of the patients developed very serious dyskinesias. Since those trials used outdated methods for cell therapy, combined with patient differences any difference in average improvement was obscured [31]. Therefore, a new trial is now planned to be conducted in Europe, in collaboration with colleagues from the United States. Since neurotransplantation might solve the problem by replacing the lost cells, further investigations in this field are justified, and are discussed in more detail in a parallel report in this issue [50].

Ablative Procedures

Thalamotomy

Stereotactic thalamotomy for Parkinson's disease was first introduced by Cooper and Hassler [13, 26]. Since then, stereotactic lesions of the ventrolateral (VL) and ventrointermedius (VIM) nuclei of the thalamus have been performed to improve medically intractable tremor in PD [16, 20, 32]; for further historical details see also Nikkhah 2011 [49]. Thalamotomy has been demonstrated to improve contralateral tremor in 45–92 % of PD patients, especially when microelectroding recording techniques for precise target localisation were used [10, 32].

In these patients, rigidity improves to a much lesser degree. Furthermore, complications have been reported in 0.5–26 % of patients, with a mortality rate ranging from 0.4 to 6 % [20, 27]. Bilateral thalamotomy, although showing a marked improvement of symptoms, carries a high risk of permanent morbidity such as speech and cognitive disturbances in about 30–50 % of the patients [63]. Thus, bilateral lesioning of the thalamic nuclei is not recommended any more [35].

Pallidotomy

Due to the overactivity of the GPi nucleus, stereotactic lesions of the GP were introduced to restore a normal electrophysiological balance in the basal ganglia circuitry [29]. Stereotactic lesions of the GPi have been demonstrated to improve both hypokinetic and hyperkinetic symptoms [29, 39]. Pallidotomy may improve up to 50 % of rigidity, bradykinesia, and tremor symptoms [17, 29]. With regard to levodopa-induced dyskinesias, pallidotomy has also shown a large therapeutic effect [39]. Furthermore, positron emission tomography (PET) studies have revealed augmentation of cortical activity, especially in the supplementary motor area (SMA) and dorsolateral prefrontal cortex, following pallidotomy procedures [11, 42, 56]. On the other hand, axial symptoms such as postural instability and gait impairment were less affected [46, 47]. Postoperative complications are usually related to the irritation or lesion of the optical tract or internal capsule due to their proximity to the posteroventral region of the GPi nucleus [39]. Permanent complication rate is estimated to be around 3.2 %, ranging from 1 to 8 %, with a 2 % mortality risk [29]. In comparison to bilateral thalamotomy, bilateral pallidotomy has been successfully performed with lower morbidity, but still with some risk of cognitive impairment [21, 29].

Lesioning the Subthalamic Nucleus

Clinical trials on STN lesions have been performed rarely due to the risk of irreversible dyskinesias [23, 30, 41, 51]. Accidentally, subthalamic nucleus lesions in PD patients due to infarctions or hemorrhages showed improvements of parkinsonian symptoms without causing dyskinesias such as hemichorea or ballism [59, 66]. Guridi and Obeso (1997) reported preliminary results of a first experience with five patients with severe PD who were submitted to a thermolytic unilateral lesion of the STN [23]. There was a significant improvement in the main parkinsonian symptoms with almost complete disappearance of gait-freezing and tremor. One out of five patients presented postoperative choreatic movements, which improved 6 months after surgery [23].

Neuromodulation (DBS)

Chronic DBS has been performed over the last 20 years to treat parkinsonian symptoms such as tremor, akinesia, rigidity, and dyskinesias in selected patients who have failed medical management [33]. Depending on the predominant parkinsonian symptoms, three different targets are available (VIM, GPi and, most frequently, STN) [3].

Experimental and clinical trials have shown that DBS using high frequencies (over 100 Hz) provide the same effects as ablative procedures, probably through a depolarisation blockade of the neuronal electrical activity of stimulated cells or axons, inducing a functional arrest or, at least, a reduction of the neuronal firing rate in the vicinity of the electrode placement [48, 52].

Post-mortem histological studies depicted a minimal lesion effect at the site of chronic stimulation and a mild surrounding gliosis, underpinning the hypothesis that the stimulation effect on clinical symptoms is least likely to be secondary to the lesion caused by the electrode placement [9].

VIM DBS

DBS of the thalamus is most often done on the VIM nucleus [5, 35, 63]. Parkinsonian patients, 70 years of age or older, suffering predominantly from disabling tremor refractory to drug therapy are the best candidates for chronic VIM stimulation [48, 54, 60, 64].

Unilateral chronic VIM stimulation showed complete tremor suppression in about 60 % of the patients and a significant improvement in 75–88 % of the cases [4, 7, 34]. Reduction of the amount of dopamine drug intake was achieved in only 15 % of the patients, as shown in long-term follow-up studies [4, 34]. Recent data showed that the best clinical effect on tremor was within the subthalamic area (STA) covering the posterior Zona incerta and prelemniscal radiation [28].

Minor postoperative side effects (dysarthria, dysequilibrium and paresthesias) from unilateral VIM stimulation may affect almost two-thirds of the patients [7]. Side- effects are well-tolerated, and disappear by turning off or just reducing stimulation voltage in most patients [6, 8]. Bilateral VIM DBS, as opposed to bilateral thalamotomy, has been shown to be safe and is not associated with a significant increase of postoperative speech and/or cognitive impairments [6, 34, 65].

In summary, VIM DBS in elderly patients with a stable and tremor dominant PD syndrome with only minor progress of off-symptoms might be the better choice compared to GPI or STN.

GPI DBS

Deep brain stimulation of the GPi is used in PD patients since 1994. Compared to VIM DBS, all PD symptoms are improved, including rigor and akinesia, reducing the mean time of the patients in "off" (from 39 to 29 %) and increasing the time spend in "on" (from 21 to 65 %) [53, 63].

The most significant effect of GIP DBS in PD patients is reduction of levodopa-induced dyskinesia by 70–90 %. Long-term follow-up showed a decrease of the effect on bradykinesia, gait, and postural stability after 3 years, and another decrease at 5 years [68]. Those patients receiving an additional STN DBS again improved their motor score. The risk of side-effects compared with bilateral pallidotomy (e.g., cognitive and speech impairments) [21, 39] is very low.

Overall, GPI DBS seems to be preferable for that group of PD patients with severe levodopa-induced dyskinesias and less severe off-symptoms.

STN DBS

Experimental studies with animal models of PD (MPTP-monkey and 6-OHDA rodent models) have demonstrated the importance of the STN in the pathophysiology of Parkinson's disease [22, 47]. Hyperactivity of the STN neurons, due to its disinhibition caused by nigrostriatal dopamine depletion, seems to be one of the major electrophysiological changes leading to an imbalance in the basal ganglia circuitry [12, 14].

Electrophysiological studies in animals depicted that STN stimulation lead to an increase on the ventromedial thalamic nucleus (Vm) electrical firing activity, probably by inhibition of the STN neuronal activity and by decreasing inhibitory activity from the SNr towards the Vm due to the reduction of SNr tonic excitation by the STN electrical blockade [22]. Improvement of thalamic activity and therefore increased stimulation of glutamatergic thalamo-cortical projections may be responsible for the improvement of hypokinetic symptoms in PD patients with STN DBS [22].

Chronic bilateral STN stimulation has been shown to improve significantly the motor function of PD patients with a stable long-term effect [2, 15, 36, 37, 58, 69]. In a prospective, randomized-pairs trial [15], patients with advanced PD underwent bilateral STN DBS and were compared to medical treatment alone. In this study, it was possible to demonstrate for the first time that not only the patients in the surgical group improved significantly with regard to motor deficits (UPDRS-III 48.0–28.3 at 6 months in the DBS group compared to 46.8–46.0 at 6 months in the BMT group) but also with regard to quality of life (PDQ-38) (DBS group: 41.8–31.8 at 6 months, BMT group 39.6–40.2 at 6 months), equal to an improvement of nearly 25 % in the DBS patients. The effect of DBS on cognitive functions and its psychiatric side-effects was assessed in an ancillary protocol as part of this randomized study [70]. In summary, STN DBS did not reduce overall cognition or affectivity, although there is a selective decrease in frontal cognitive functions and an improvement in anxiety in patients after the treatment. None of these changes affected improvements in quality of life.

Gait and axial symptoms demonstrate a better improvement after bilateral STN stimulation compared to unilateral stimulation [44]. On the other hand, STN stimulation may not directly improve dyskinesias, but indirectly due to the reduction of the daily drug dose [38, 43, 63]. Reduction of the dose of L-dopa medication may range from 30 to 50 % of the preoperative doses [38, 43].

Abnormal involuntary movements such as dyskinesias, ballism, and chorea are the most frequent side-effects related to STN stimulation [45, 63]. Nevertheless, reduction in the intensity of the stimulation usually eliminates or diminishes abnormal movements [45, 63].

Comparison between pallidal and STN chronic bilateral stimulation, bradykinesia, akinesia, and general movements shows a better rate of recovery following DBS in the STN, and additionally, cortical activation is clearly more pronounced in patients submitted to DBS of the STN compared to those that underwent Gpi DBS [42]. Furthermore, reduction in the daily drug doses in PD patients following bilateral STN stimulation seems to be more pronounced compared to patients treated with GPi stimulation [38, 42], although this has been challenged in more recent studies [19]. There are also some clear limitations with STN DBS, such as the lack of clinical improvement of gait and balance in PD patients [67].

Conclusion

Neurosurgical treatment strategies for Parkinson's disease have changed dramatically within the last 40 years, based on the increase in the scientific and clinical knowledge of underlying pathological, pathophysiological, and plasticity mechanisms determining the course of the disease [61]. Progressive nigrostriatal degeneration in Parkinson's disease has now been related to different mechanisms [1, 24, 40].

Deep-brain stimulation has been shown to be effective with regard to significant improvement on the motor scales in the surgical group vs best medical treatment [15] in selected PD patients. Furthermore, quality of life was significantly improved with regard to the PDQ-39 summary index as well as several subscores, e.g., activities of daily living or emotional well-being. Psychiatric and neuropsychological side-effects, which were part of an ancillary protocol, showed no reduction of overall cognition and affectivity [70]. Three different targets are suitable for PD patients, depending on the clinical presentation. Since STN alleviates all symptoms, this target seems to be the most frequently used one. VIM might be indicated in elderly PD patients with a mainly tremor-dominant PD, GPi in patients with severe levodopa induced dyskinesias. In our experience, lesioning in PD patients is less frequently performed nowadays, at least in Western countries. Exemptions might be a unilateral thalamotomy in a unilateral, tremor-dominant elderly PD patient. The significance of cell-based therapies, in contrast, has still to be fully evaluated. Taken together, neurosurgical treatment strategies such as DBS and lesioning play in important role in today's management of PD patients, whereas more novel therapies such as stem-cell transplantation and gene therapy hold great potential for the future.

Acknowledgements Parts of this study have been supported by grants from the Weber Petri Foundation and the German Parkinson Foundation.

Conflict of Interest Drs. Pinsker and Nikkhah report having received speaking fees from Medtronic. Dr. Nikkhah has also served as a Consultant for Medtronic. No other potential conflict of interest relevant to this article was reported.

References

1. Ben Shlomo Y (1997) The epidemiology of Parkinson's disease. Baillieres Clin Neurol 6:55–68
2. Benabid AL, Chabardes S, Mitrofanis J, Pollak P (2009) Deep brain stimulation of the subthalamic nucleus for the treatment of Parkinson's disease. Lancet Neurol 8:67–81

3. Benabid AL, Benazzouz A, Hoffmann D, Limousin P, Krack P, Pollak P (1998) Long-term electrical inhibition of deep brain targets in movement disorders. Mov Disord 13(Suppl 3):119–125
4. Benabid AL, Pollak P, Gao D, Hoffmann D, Limousin P, Gay E, Payen I, Benazzouz A (1996) Chronic electrical stimulation of the ventralis intermedius nucleus of the thalamus as a treatment of movement disorders. J Neurosurg 84:203–214
5. Benabid AL, Pollak P, Gervason C, Hoffmann D, Gao DM, Hommel M, Perret JE, de Rougemont J (1991) Long-term suppression of tremor by chronic stimulation of the ventral intermediate thalamic nucleus. Lancet 337:403–406
6. Benabid AL, Pollak P, Louveau A, Henry S, de Rougemont J (1987) Combined (thalamotomy and stimulation) stereotactic surgery of the VIM thalamic nucleus for bilateral Parkinson disease. Appl Neurophysiol 50:344–346
7. Blond S, Caparros-Lefebvre D, Parker F, Assaker R, Petit H, Guieu JD, Christiaens JL (1992) Control of tremor and involuntary movement disorders by chronic stereotactic stimulation of the ventral intermediate thalamic nucleus. J Neurosurg 77:62–68
8. Burleigh AL, Horak FB, Burchiel KJ, Nutt JG (1993) Effects of thalamic stimulation on tremor, balance, and step initiation: a single subject study. Mov Disord 8:519–524
9. Caparros-Lefebvre D, Ruchoux MM, Blond S, Petit H, Percheron G (1994) Long-term thalamic stimulation in Parkinson's disease: postmortem anatomoclinical study. Neurology 44:1856–1860
10. Cardoso F, Jankovic J, Grossman RG, Hamilton WJ (1995) Outcome after stereotactic thalamotomy for dystonia and hemiballismus. Neurosurgery 36:501–507
11. Ceballos-Baumann AO, Obeso JA, Vitek JL, DeLong MR, Bakay R, Linazasoro G, Brooks DJ (1994) Restoration of thalamocortical activity after posteroventral pallidotomy in Parkinson's disease. Lancet 344:814
12. Chevalier G, Deniau JM (1990) Disinhibition as a basic process in the expression of striatal functions. Trends Neurosci 13:277–280
13. Cooper IS (1956) Neurosurgical alleviation of parkinsonism. Am Surg 22:1070–1075
14. DeLong MR (1990) Primate models of movement disorders of basal ganglia origin. Trends Neurosci 13:281–285
15. Deuschl G, Schade-Brittinger C, Krack P, Volkmann J, Schafer H, Botzel K, Daniels C, Deutschlander A, Dillmann U, Eisner W, Gruber D, Hamel W, Herzog J, Hilker R, Klebe S, Kloss M, Koy J, Krause M, Kupsch A, Lorenz D, Lorenzl S, Mehdorn HM, Moringlane JR, Oertel W, Pinsker MO, Reichmann H, Reuss A, Schneider GH, Schnitzler A, Steude U, Sturm V, Timmermann L, Tronnier V, Trottenberg T, Wojtecki L, Wolf E, Poewe W, Voges J (2006) A randomized trial of deep-brain stimulation for Parkinson's disease. N Engl J Med 355:896–908
16. Diederich NJ, Alesch F (1997) Neurosurgical methods in treatment of Parkinson disease. Current status. Nervenarzt 68:466–476
17. Dogali M, Fazzini E, Kolodny E, Eidelberg D, Sterio D, Devinsky O, Beric A (1995) Stereotactic ventral pallidotomy for Parkinson's disease. Neurology 45:753–761
18. Duvoisin RC (1992) A brief history of parkinsonism. Neurol Clin 10:301–316
19. Evidente VG, Prekumar AP, Adler CH, Caviness JN, Driver-Dunckley E, Lyons MK (2011) Medication dose reductions after pallidal versus subthalamic stimulation in patients with Parkinson's disease. Acta Neurol Scand 124(3):211–214
20. Fox MW, Ahlskog JE, Kelly PJ (1991) Stereotactic ventrolateralis thalamotomy for medically refractory tremor in post-levodopa era Parkinson's disease patients. J Neurosurg 75:723–730
21. Galvez-Jimenez N, Lozano A, Tasker R, Duff J, Hutchison W, Lang AE (1998) Pallidal stimulation in Parkinson's disease patients with a prior unilateral pallidotomy. Can J Neurol Sci 25:300–305
22. Gao D, Benazzouz A, Bressand K, Piallat B, Benabid AL (1997) Roles of GABA, glutamate, acetylcholine and STN stimulation on thalamic VM in rats. Neuroreport 8:2601–2605
23. Guridi J, Obeso JA (1997) The role of the subthalamic nucleus in the origin of hemiballism and parkinsonism: new surgical perspectives. Adv Neurol 74:235–247
24. Halliday G, Lees A, Stern M (2011) Milestones in Parkinson's disease – clinical and pathologic features. Mov Disord 26:1015–1021
25. Hassani OK, Mouroux M, Feger J (1996) Increased subthalamic neuronal activity after nigral dopaminergic lesion independent of disinhibition via the globus pallidus. Neuroscience 72:105–115
26. Hassler R, Riechert T, Mundinger F, Umbach W, Ganglberger JA (1960) Physiological observations in stereotaxic operations in extrapyramidal motor disturbances. Brain 83:337–350
27. Hauser R, Freeman T, Olanow C (1995) Surgical therapies for Parkinson's disease. In: Kurlan R (ed) Treatment of movement disorders. J. B. Lippincott Company, Philadelphia, pp 57–93
28. Herzog J, Hamel W, Wenzelburger R, Potter M, Pinsker MO, Bartussek J, Morsnowski A, Steigerwald F, Deuschl G, Volkmann J (2007) Kinematic analysis of thalamic versus subthalamic neurostimulation in postural and intention tremor. Brain 130:1608–1625
29. Iacono RP, Shima F, Lonser RR, Kuniyoshi S, Maeda G, Yamada S (1995) The results, indications, and physiology of posteroventral pallidotomy for patients with Parkinson's disease. Neurosurgery 36:1118–1125
30. Inzelberg R, Korczyn AD (1994) Persistent hemiballism in Parkinson's disease. J Neurol Neurosurg Psychiatry 57:1013–1014
31. Isacson O (2009) Cell therapy ahead for Parkinson's disease. Science 326:1060
32. Jankovic J, Cardoso F, Grossman RG, Hamilton WJ (1995) Outcome after stereotactic thalamotomy for parkinsonian, essential, and other types of tremor. Neurosurgery 37:680–686
33. Kleiner-Fisman G, Herzog J, Fisman DN, Tamma F, Lyons KE, Pahwa R, Lang AE, Deuschl G (2006) Subthalamic nucleus deep brain stimulation: summary and meta-analysis of outcomes. Mov Disord 21(Suppl 14):S290–S304
34. Koller W, Pahwa R, Busenbark K, Hubble J, Wilkinson S, Lang A, Tuite P, Sime E, Lazano A, Hauser R, Malapira T, Smith D, Tarsy D, Miyawaki E, Norregaard T, Kormos T, Olanow CW (1997) High-frequency unilateral thalamic stimulation in the treatment of essential and parkinsonian tremor. Ann Neurol 42:292–299
35. Koller W, Wilkinson S, Pahwa R et al (1998) Surgical treatment options in Parkinson's disease. In: Bakay R (ed) Neurosurgery Clinics of North America: surgical treatment movement disorders. W. B. Saunders Company, Philadelphia, pp 295–306
36. Krack P, Batir A, Van Blercom N, Chabardes S, Fraix V, Ardouin C, Koudsie A, Limousin PD, Benazzouz A, LeBas JF, Benabid AL, Pollak P (2003) Five-year follow-up of bilateral stimulation of the subthalamic nucleus in advanced Parkinson's disease. N Engl J Med 349:1925–1934
37. Krack P, Limousin P, Benabid AL, Pollak P (1997) Chronic stimulation of subthalamic nucleus improves levodopa-induced dyskinesias in Parkinson's disease. Lancet 350:1676
38. Krack P, Pollak P, Limousin P, Hoffmann D, Benazzouz A, Le Bas JF, Koudsie A, Benabid AL (1998) Opposite motor effects of pallidal stimulation in Parkinson's disease. Ann Neurol 43:180–192
39. Laitinen LV, Bergenheim AT, Hariz MI (1992) Leksell's Posteroventral pallidotomy in the treatment of Parkinson's disease. J Neurosurg 76:53–61
40. Lang AE, Lozano AM (1998) Parkinson's disease. First of two parts. N Engl J Med 339:1044–1053
41. Lee MS, Marsden CD (1994) Movement disorders following lesions of the thalamus or subthalamic region. Mov Disord 9:493–507
42. Limousin P, Greene J, Pollak P, Rothwell J, Benabid AL, Frackowiak R (1997) Changes in cerebral activity pattern due to subthalamic nucleus or internal pallidum stimulation in Parkinson's disease. Ann Neurol 42:283–291
43. Limousin P, Krack P, Pollak P, Benazzouz A, Ardouin C, Hoffmann D, Benabid AL (1998) Electrical stimulation of the subthalamic nucleus in advanced Parkinson's disease. N Engl J Med 339:1105–1111

44. Limousin P, Pollak P, Benazzouz A, Hoffmann D, Le Bas JF, Broussolle E, Perret JE, Benabid AL (1995) Effect of parkinsonian signs and symptoms of bilateral subthalamic nucleus stimulation. Lancet 345:91–95
45. Limousin P, Pollak P, Hoffmann D, Benazzouz A, Perret JE, Benabid AL (1996) Abnormal involuntary movements induced by subthalamic nucleus stimulation in parkinsonian patients. Mov Disord 11:231–235
46. Lozano AM, Lang AE, Galvez-Jimenez N, Miyasaki J, Duff J, Hutchinson WD, Dostrovsky JO (1995) Effect of GPi pallidotomy on motor function in Parkinson's disease. Lancet 346:1383–1387
47. Lozano A, Lang A (1998) Pallidotomy for Parkinson's disease. In: Bakay R (ed) Neurosurgery Clinics of North America: surgical treatment of movement disorders. W. B. Saunders Company, Philadelphia, pp 325–336
48. Mendis T, Suchowersky O, Lang A, Gauthier S (1999) Management of Parkinson's disease a review of current and new therapies. Can J Neurol Sci 26:89–103
49. Nikkhah G (2011) Journeys to the center of the brain. 60 years of stereotactic neurosurgery at the University Hospital Freiburg. Nikkhah G, Freiburg
50. Nikkhah G (2013) Restorative strategies for the dopaminergic nigrostriatal projection pathway. In: Nikkhah G, Pinsker M (eds) Stereotactic and Functional Neurosurgery. Acta Neurochirurgica Suppl. Springer, Wien, pp 79–85
51. Obeso JA, Guridi J, Linazasoro G, Ramos E (1995) Hemiballism in Parkinson's disease. J Neurol Neurosurg Psychiatry 58:645–647
52. Obeso JA, Rodriguez MC, Gorospe A, Guridi J, Alvarez L, Macias R (1997) Surgical treatment of Parkinson's disease. Baillieres Clin Neurol 6:125–145
53. Pahwa R, Wilkinson S, Smith D, Lyons K, Miyawaki E, Koller WC (1997) High-frequency stimulation of the globus pallidus for the treatment of Parkinson's disease. Neurology 49:249–253
54. Pollak P, Benabid AL, Gross C, Gao DM, Laurent A, Benazzouz A, Hoffmann D, Gentil M, Perret J (1993) Effects of the stimulation of the subthalamic nucleus in Parkinson disease. Rev Neurol (Paris) 149:175–176
55. Quinn N (1997) Parkinson's disease: clinical features. In: Quinn N (ed) Clinical neurology. Parkinsonism. Bailliere Tindall, London, pp 1–13
56. Samuel M, Ceballos-Baumann AO, Turjanski N, Boecker H, Gorospe A, Linazasoro G, Holmes AP, DeLong MR, Vitek JL, Thomas DG, Quinn NP, Obeso JA, Brooks DJ (1997) Pallidotomy in Parkinson's disease increases supplementary motor area and prefrontal activation during performance of volitional movements an H2(15)O PET study. Brain 120(Pt 8):1301–1313
57. Schapira A (1997) Pathogenesis of Parkinson's disease. In: Quinn N (ed) Clinical neurology. International practice and research. Parkinsonism. Bailliere Tindall, London, pp 15–36
58. Schupbach WM, Chastan N, Welter ML, Houeto JL, Mesnage V, Bonnet AM, Czernecki V, Maltete D, Hartmann A, Mallet L, Pidoux B, Dormont D, Navarro S, Cornu P, Mallet A, Agid Y (2005) Stimulation of the subthalamic nucleus in Parkinson's disease: a 5 year follow up. J Neurol Neurosurg Psychiatry 76:1640–1644
59. Sellal F, Hirsch E, Lisovoski F, Mutschler V, Collard M, Marescaux C (1992) Contralateral disappearance of parkinsonian signs after subthalamic hematoma. Neurology 42:255–256
60. Siegfried J, Lippitz B (1994) Bilateral chronic electrostimulation of ventroposterolateral pallidum: a new therapeutic approach for alleviating all parkinsonian symptoms. Neurosurgery 35:1126–1129
61. Smith ID, Grace AA (1992) Role of the subthalamic nucleus in the regulation of nigral dopamine neuron activity. Synapse 12: 287–303
62. Spiegel EA, Wycis HT, Marks M, Lee AJ (1947) Stereotaxic apparatus for operations on the human brain. Science 106:349–350
63. Starr PA, Vitek JL, Bakay RA (1998) Deep brain stimulation for movement disorders. Neurosurg Clin N Am 9:381–402
64. Strafella A, Ashby P, Munz M, Dostrovsky JO, Lozano AM, Lang AE (1997) Inhibition of voluntary activity by thalamic stimulation in humans: relevance for the control of tremor. Mov Disord 12:727–737
65. Tsubokawa T, Katayama Y, Yamamoto T (1995) Control of persistent hemiballismus by chronic thalamic stimulation. Report of two cases. J Neurosurg 82:501–505
66. Vidakovic A, Dragasevic N, Kostic VS (1994) Hemiballism: report of 25 cases. J Neurol Neurosurg Psychiatry 57:945–949
67. Vingerhoets FJ, Tagliati M (2012) Treating PD axial signs with DBS: is two better than one? Neurology 78:1036–1037
68. Volkmann J, Allert N, Voges J, Sturm V, Schnitzler A, Freund HJ (2004) Long-term results of bilateral pallidal stimulation in Parkinson's disease. Ann Neurol 55:871–875
69. Weaver F, Follett K, Hur K, Ippolito D, Stern M (2005) Deep brain stimulation in Parkinson disease: a metaanalysis of patient outcomes. J Neurosurg 103:956–967
70. Witt K, Daniels C, Reiff J, Krack P, Volkmann J, Pinsker MO, Krause M, Tronnier V, Kloss M, Schnitzler A, Wojtecki L, Botzel K, Danek A, Hilker R, Sturm V, Kupsch A, Karner E, Deuschl G (2008) Neuropsychological and psychiatric changes after deep brain stimulation for Parkinson's disease: a randomised, multicentre study. Lancet Neurol 7:605–614

Improving MRT Image Quality in Patients with Movement Disorders

Elisabeth Schültke, Norbert Nanko, Marcus Pinsker, Michael Katzev, Alexandra Sebastian, Bernd Feige, and Guido Nikkhah

Abstract *Objective*: In order to improve image quality in a simultaneous fMRI-EEG study with patients suffering from the involuntary movements typical for Huntington's disease, the aim was to develop a technique for immobilizing the heads of our patients inside an MRI head coil.

Methods: We modified a mask technique previously used for reliable repositioning in temporally fractionated radiotherapy. The mask was tested in three patients with Huntington's disease, acquiring structural and functional MR images with simultaneous EEG with and without the mask.

Results: Image as well as EEG signal quality were significantly improved in patients wearing the mask. However, the image quality with mask was comparable to acquisitions from patients without movement disorders only in patients with light to moderate dyskinesia. Although image quality was also significantly improved in a patient suffering from severe dyskinesia with quasi-continuous involuntary movements, the quality of both the MR images as well as the EEG signal was lower than what would be expected in a healthy control person.

Conclusion: We have succeeded in developing a mask that fits into the MRI head coil, does not disturb the MRI signal, and significantly improves both fMRI and EEG signal quality.

Keywords fMRI • Dyskinesia • EEG • Huntington's disease • Immobilization • Mask

Introduction

Because of the choreatic movements typical for patients with Huntington's disease, it is extremely difficult to obtain high quality images of the intracranial structures. When we started a new study with the aim of correlating tests to assess our patients' impulse control behavior with simultaneous EEG and fMRI, data from only one out of eight Huntington patients with mild to moderate chorea who underwent functional magnetic resonance imaging (fMRI) were of sufficient

E. Schültke, MD, PhD (✉)
Division of Stereotactic and Functional Neurosurgery, Department of General Neurosurgery, University Medical Center Freiburg, Breisacher Straße 64, Freiburg D-79106, Germany
e-mail: elisabeth.schueltke@uniklinik-freiburg.de

N. Nanko
Department of Radiooncology, Neurocentre, Albert-Ludwigs-University, Freiburg, Germany

M. Pinsker, MD
Division of Stereotactic and Functional Neurosurgery, Department of General Neurosurgery, Neurosurgical Clinic, University Medical Center Freiburg, Breisacher Straße 64, Freiburg D-79106, Germany

Klinik für Neurochirurgie, HELIOS Klinikum Berlin-Buch, Schwanebecker Chaussee 50, Berlin DE-13125, Germany

M. Katzev
Department of Neurology, Neurocentre, Albert-Ludwigs-University, Freiburg, Germany

A. Sebastian and B. Feige
Department of Psychiatry and Psychotherapy, Neurocentre, Albert-Ludwigs-University, Freiburg, Germany

G. Nikkhah, MD, PhD
Division of Stereotactic and Functional Neurosurgery, Department of General Neurosurgery, Neurosurgical Clinic, University Medical Center Freiburg, Breisacher Straße 64, Freiburg D-79106, Germany

Neurosurgical Clinic, University Hospital Erlangen, Schwabachanlage 6, Erlangen D-91054, Germany
e-mail: guido.nikkhah@uk-erlangen.de

Electronic supplementary material
The online version of this chapter (doi:10.1007/978-3-7091-1482-7_3) contains supplementary material, which is available to authorized users.

Elisabeth Schültke and Norbert Nanko have contributed equally to the work described in this manuscript.

quality to be included in the study. The remainder of the data had to be discarded because of extensive movement artifacts. At this point, we decided to develop an external fixation device for the head, in order to restrict involuntary movements. Our device used a shell-type head mold and a face mask, both fitted individually for each patient, similar to the immobilization devices used in fractionated radiotherapy. Our device is fast and easy to produce, and fits into the head coil of a 3T MRI scanner (Magnetom Trio, Siemens).

Materials and Methods

To develop the immobilization device and test its efficiency, one healthy volunteer and three patients with Huntington's disease were recruited. While the basic production principle was similar to that for the devices routinely fitted for patients who undergo fractionated stereotactic radiosurgery, we had to adapt both the production process and the final product to the unique requirements of our purpose. Those requirements were the following:

1. The patient's head covered with the EEG cap should fit snugly inside the mask, which in turn should fit snugly inside the MRI head coil in order to prevent or at least significantly reduce the extent of sudden involuntary movements, yet without causing undue claustrophobia or even pressure sores.
2. The patient's head should be in a position that allows him or her to see the mirrored computer screen with the fMRI tasks.
3. The entire setup should be sufficiently comfortable over a period of at least 45 min, so as not to distract the patient from the tasks.

Recruitment and testing were conducted according to the rules of the Ethics Committee at the University Hospital in Freiburg, Germany. All test subjects signed informed consent for all components of the test procedure.

Immobilization Device Fitting in the MRI Head Coil

Mask development was conducted in one healthy volunteer. The mask was produced in two parts: one face mask and one occipital half-shell (head mold) for positioning of the back of the head as well as most of the neck. The exact fit of the face mask with the occipital half-shell is guaranteed by the unique 3D mask geometry. Measurements were taken of the 3T Siemens MRI head coil, and a mould was fabricated from NECURON® 600 (Necumer-Product GmbH, Bohmte, Germany), a low density and high durability casting material, as shown in Fig. 1a. Also based on the measurements of the MRI head coil, a special horseshoe-shaped holder was constructed from plexiglass and steel bolts, as shown in Fig. 1b. This holder supports the back of the patient's head in such a position that it will later fit the occipital half shell, while at the same time the patient is still able to see the mirrored computer screen with the test tasks.

As a first step in the actual fitting process, the EEG electrode cap is placed on the patient's head. The patient is asked to lie down in supine position, with the head on the horseshoe-shaped holder, and to fixate a point on the ceiling exactly overhead. Out of four equally shaped but differently sized support pillows (produced in the workshop of the Department of Radiotherapy), the one that fits the patient's neck most comfortably is chosen. The patient is asked to sit up again.

Next, the occipital half-shell is produced. One 3-mm-thick non-perforated, 30×45 cm thermoplastic sheet (TURBOCAST®, Essenzia Medical, Freiburg, Germany) is warmed in a 65 °C water bath until malleable and then placed on top of the plexiglass horseshoe, where it is fixed with the help of four fastening clamps. The patient is again asked to lie down with the back of the head inside the horseshoe, stretching the TURBOCAST® sheet gently but steadily. From below, both the TURBOCAST® sheet and the patient's head are supported by the two cupped hands of an assistant. At this point, pressurized air is used to speed the cooling process of the material. Once cooled down, the material is not malleable any more.

In the next step, with the patient still lying on the back, the face mask is produced from a 2-mm-thick perforated TURBOCAST® sheet, also 30 × 45 cm. After a thin cotton veil is placed on the patient's face, the thermoplastic sheet is placed to cover the entire face, care being taken to tightly fit prominent landmarks like the orbital ridges, bridge of the nose and chin, as well as the frontal and lateral electrodes in the EEG cap.

Pressurized air is again used to speed the cooling process of the material. Before the mask material is removed, the shape of the eyes is marked with the help of a small template. A short break follows during which the patient is asked to sit upright without disturbing the fit of the EEG cap.

The mould shown in Fig. 1 is now covered with a thin plastic film; the occipital half shell is fitted into it, and the space in-between is filled with B45, a 2-component polyurethane foam (Von Corvin, Hamburg, Germany). Since the foam develops considerably high temperatures during its hardening process, pressurized air is used to cool the foam for about 10 min in order to prevent the occipital shell from softening and losing its shape (Fig. 1c). Once the foam is hardened, any surplus material is sawed off and the edges are sanded. Hollows for the eyes and nostrils are cut out of the face mask; the edges of the holes are covered with tape to soften them and to prevent irritation of the patient's skin.

A strip of Velcro of about 5 cm is glued on the facing right and left sides of occipital shell and face mask, in order to allow a tight fit around the patient's head. The patient is asked to lie down in the mould with the occipital shell (Fig. 1d, e). A mark to indicate the preferred position of the eyebrow (in the same position where this marker is found on the MRI head coil) serves as landmark for the assessment of

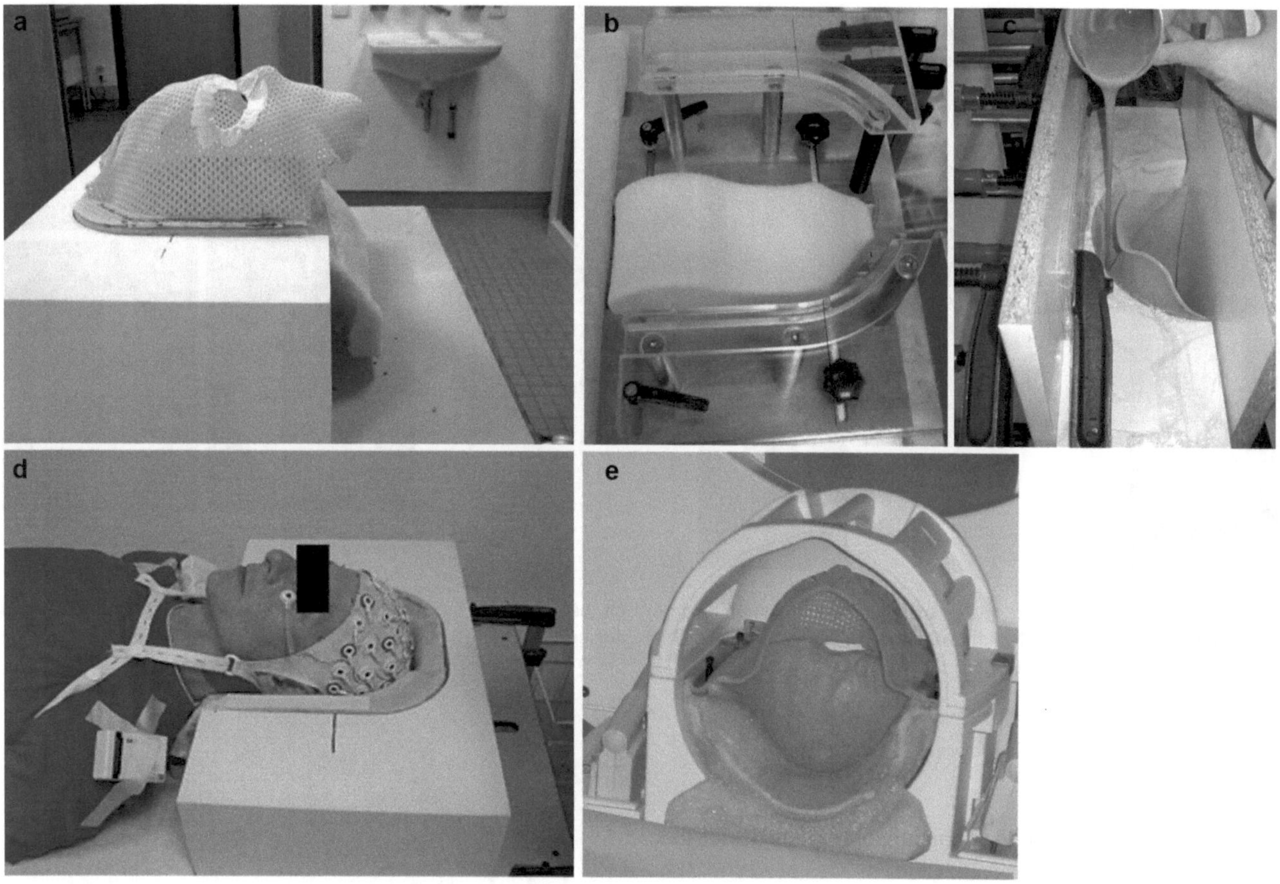

Fig. 1 Production of the immobilization device. Positioning device composed of shell and face mask in the NECURON® mold (**a**). The size of the mold is identical to that of the MRI coil and the *broken black line* on the mold represents the marking for the eye brow position on the coil. Plexiglass holder for correct neck position (**b**). Production of the occipital shell (**c**). Test for fit of the mask in the MRI mold (**d**) and in the MRI coil (**e**)

good patient positioning. In the case that there is no good fit, the mask production procedure needs to be repeated. With good fit, the patient can proceed to the MRI department. A video of 5 min length showing the mask production in greater detail has been produced (Video 1). It will take two persons between 1.5 and 2 h to produce the mask, amounting to a total of four person hours. The additional costs for materials are about 100 Euro.

Our tests, using a phantom first followed by testing the healthy volunteer with the fixation device in the MRI, showed that there were no signal interferences from the mask material. Image analysis was controlled for artifacts, and direct contrast was used with and without mask.

Quality Test for Immobilization in Three Patients with Huntington's Disease

Of the three patients tested, two had mild to moderate chorea (2 and 10 points on the Unified Huntington's Disease Rating Scale (UHDRS) category 12) and reached total UHDRS motor scores of 16 and 29 respectively; one patient suffered from strong chorea (15 points in UHDRS category 12) and was assigned an UHDRS score of 34. In one of the patients with light to moderate dyskinesia, we had already attempted to acquire fMRI several months earlier. However, the quality of the obtained images was poor due to multiple movement artifacts, and they had to be excluded from the intended fMRI study. The extent of continuous dyskinesia of the neck musculature in the third patient would have prevented even the attempt of MR imaging before the immobilization device became available. All three patients had a mask fitted as described above.

For each patient, the duration of the fMRI session was about 45 min. Simultaneous EEG was acquired via 64 surface electrodes. In addition, a set of anatomical T1 images (MPRAGE) was acquired. For this acquisition, the EEG cap was removed to avoid MR signal disturbance and possible electrode heating. In order to fill the space of the now-removed EEG cap, a thin flannel sheet was placed between the patient's head and the occipital shell.

Data analysis was conducted using SPM 5 (Wellcome Department of Cognitive Neurology), running with Matlab 7.7.0 (The Mathworks Inc., Natick, MA, USA) for the MR images and avg_q (Dr. Bernd Feige, Freiburg; https://github.com/berndf/avg_q) for the EEG signals.

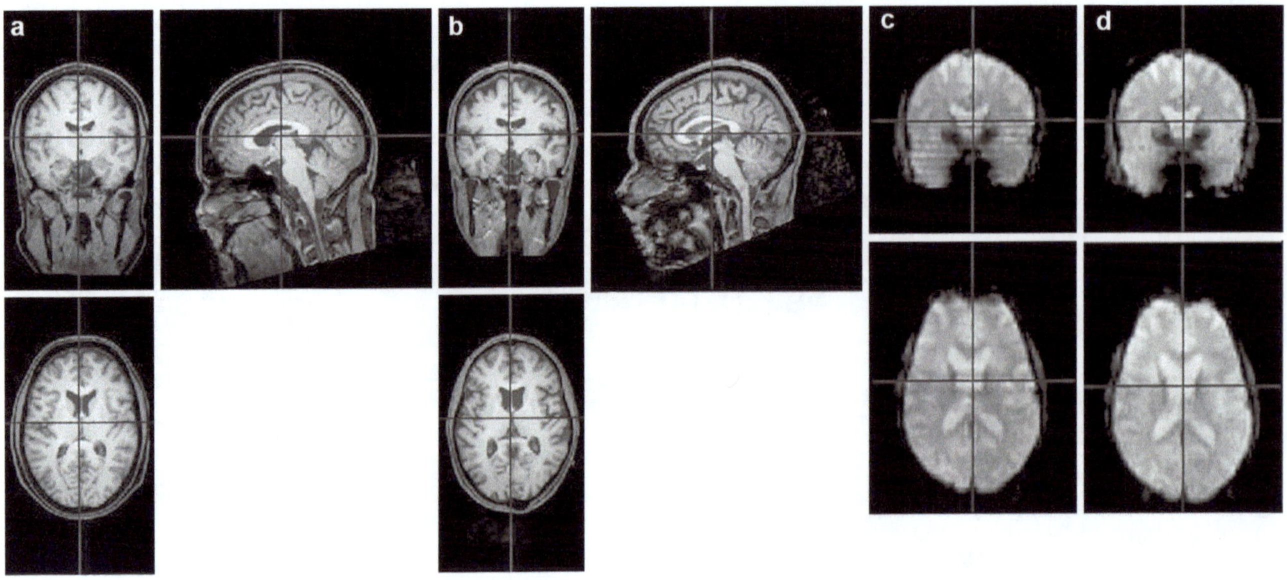

Fig. 2 Improvement of image quality with the immobilization device. Coronal and axial images of healthy volunteer (**a**) and patient (**b**). T2*-weighted echo-planar image (EPI) of the same patient (chorea score 2) on the same day: Patient without (**c**) and with (**d**) the immobilization device

Results

We have succeeded in producing an immobilization device that fits into a commercially available Siemens MRI head coil. It is comfortable enough for the patient to wear during the about 45-min period of data acquisition. At the same time, it allows the patient to comfortably follow the test tasks presented on a computer screen mirrored inside the MRI bore. The head immobilization during the acquisition of fMRI images and simultaneously acquired EEG signals resulted in significantly improved quality in both images and EEG signals.

Improved Quality of Structural and Functional MRI Images

Structural (T1) images in patients with light to moderate chorea were similar in quality to the images obtained from the healthy volunteer (Fig. 2a, b).

The quality of functional MR images was significantly improved when the patient was scanned with his head inside the immobilization device, as compared to images acquired within an hour on the same patient but without immobilization device (Fig. 2c, d).

Improved Quality of EEG Signals

The quality of the EEG signals was significantly improved when the patients were wearing the immobilization device.

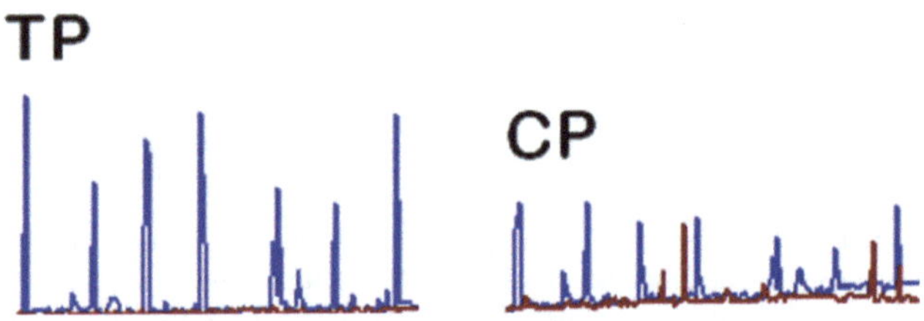

Fig. 3 Improvement of EEG signal. EEG amplitude at different positions during the Simon task in the same patient. *Blue*: Signal acquired without mask, *Red*: Signal acquired with mask

Figure 3 shows the amplitude time course of the EEG after correction for the fMRI scanning artifact for two EEG channels. The frequency of strong artifacts and also the incidence of smaller artifacts were clearly reduced by the mask.

Discussion

There have been a number of publications about attempts to reduce patient-generated movement artifacts during image acquisition. Some of the methods build on the active collaboration of the patient, while others rely on immobilization forced by external devices. Epstein reports on an interesting study conducted in children with attention-deficit/hyperactivity disorder (ADHD), where data losses due to movement artifacts were reduced from 42 % to about 10 % after behavioral training in a mock scanner unit [4]. In addition, de Bie and colleagues reported a success rate of 94 % for structural and 66 % for functional MRI in very young children after behavioural training [3]. However, in patients with movement disorders, many of the artefact-producing movements occur involuntarily, and thus are very difficult to modulate with behavioural training. This is where external devices that force immobilization could play a beneficial role. The oral lore was discouraging, because it stated that the attempt of forced head immobilization actually resulted in an increase of movement artifacts, possibly because the patients perceive the force of the immobilizing device as unpleasant and try to counteract it. However, there are reports from various groups about the use of other, external immobilization devices for imaging procedures. Bettinardi and colleagues successfully used a polyacrylic hemicylinder in combination with dental material for fixation of the teeth in CT, MRI, and PET imaging [1]. Shrawder and colleagues demonstrated that a mask system similar to ours allowed reliable repositioning with patients undergoing lengthy CT investigation [5]. Beyer demonstrated that shell-type molded head holders are more efficient in reducing movement artifacts than vacuum-lock bags [2]. The improved quality of both structural and functional images as well as of the EEG signals we observed in our patients, using a combination of personalized shell-type head mold and face mask, support this assessment. Meanwhile, we have used the mask in the assessment of eight patients with Huntington's disease. One patient with a known tendency to claustrophobic attacks asked for premature termination of the test series. The other seven patients produced a complete set of valuable data in all three categories, impulse control testing, EEG, and fMRI.

Although the incentive for our work was to improve image quality in the setting of a synchronized fMRI and EEG study, our immobilization device might prove useful also in other patients with movement disorders, where high-quality MR images of the head need to be acquired. The production process for the device is fast and reliable in experienced hands, with material costs of less than 100 Euro. It could be a valuable alternative to acquiring MR images under anesthesia to avoid movement artifacts. Especially where repeated imaging is planned in such patients, the one-time fabrication of a personalized shell-and-mask device would appear to be a sensible investment for improving image quality.

Acknowledgments We would like to thank Dipl. Physiol. Christoph Weis, who made the initial suggestion for the development of the mask, and Dr. Oliver Tüscher for encouraging us to go ahead with the idea. We also thank Mr. Kraft, Mr. Salvatore Fresta, and Mr. Benjamin Grunert of the Department of Radiotherapy for their time and enthusiasm during the development phase of our mask technique, as well as for their continued and ongoing support in fitting masks for our patients. Prof. A. Grosu, director of the Department of Radiotherapy, is thanked for allowing us to conduct this development work in the departmental workshop. EEG and fMRI data were acquired as part of a larger project supported by the Ministry of Education and Research of Germany (BMBF).

Conflict of Interest The authors declare that they have no conflict of interest.

References

1. Bettinardi V, Scardaoni R, Gilardi MC, Rizzo G, Perani D, Paulesu E, Striano G, Triluzi F, Fazio F (1991) Head holder for PET, CT and MR studies. J Comput Assist Tomogr 15(5):886–892
2. Beyer T, Tellmann L, Nickel I, Uwe Pietrzyk U (2005) On the use of positioning aids to reduce misregistration in the head and neck in whole-body PET/CT studies. J Nucl Med 46:596–602
3. de Bie HM, Boersma M, Wattjes MP, Adriaanse S, Vermeulen RJ, Oostrom KJ, Huisman J, Veltman DJ, Delemarre-Van de Waal HA (2010) Preparing children with a mock scanner training protocol results in high quality structural and functional MRI scans. Eur J Pediatr 169(9):1079–1085
4. Epstein JN, Casey BJ, Tonev ST, Davidson M, Reiss AL, Garrett A, Hinshaw SP, Greenhill LL, Vitolo A, Kotler LA, Jarrett MA, Spicer J (2007) Assessment and prevention of head motion during imaging of patients with attention deficit hyperactivity disorder. Psychiatry Res 155(1):75–82
5. Shrawder S, Lapin GD, Allen CV, Vick NA, Groothuis DR (1994) A new head holder for reducing axial movement and repositioning errors during physiological CT imaging. J Comput Assist Tomogr 18(2):329–336

STN Stimulation in General Anaesthesia: Evidence Beyond 'Evidence-Based Medicine'

Christian K.E. Moll, Sebastian Payer, Alessandro Gulberti, Andrew Sharrott, Simone Zittel, Kai Boelmans, Johannes Köppen, Christian Gerloff, Manfred Westphal, Andreas K. Engel, Christian Oehlwein, Carsten Buhmann, and Wolfgang Hamel

Abstract Awake surgery is regarded mandatory for optimal electrode implantation into the subthalamic nucleus (STN) for deep brain stimulation (DBS) in Parkinson's disease (PD). However, this is questionable since general anaesthesia (GA) does not preclude intraoperative microrecordings and clinical evaluation of, for example, current spread to the corticospinal tract. In addition, even in the awake state, clinical testing is not without limitations. We report on intra- and postoperative findings in 11 patients suffering from advanced PD who were operated under GA (propofol/remifentanil). The activity of STN neurons under GA was characterized by excessive burst discharges that differed fundamentally from the irregular tonic patterns observed in the STN of awake patients. In all patients, we obtained improved motor symptoms and reduced levodopa-induced dyskinesias and motor fluctuations, which was associated with a reduction in the levodopa equivalent daily dose. Therapeutic DBS was not limited by current spread to the corticospinal tract in any of the patients. The trajectories chosen for electrode implantation in GA compared well to awake surgery. Our results indicate that STN surgery in GA can be performed in a safe manner. It can be offered to anxious patients, and represents a viable option when awake surgery bears a risk for the patient.

Keywords Deep brain stimulation • Subthalamic nucleus • STN stimulation • Parkinson's disease • General anaesthesia • Microelectrode recordings

Introduction

It is argued that awake surgery is a prerequisite in the search for the 'optimal' target during STN electrode implantation in Parkinson's disease. This is put into perspective if we consider that the so-called 'optimal' target is merely the *best possible* target, i.e., surgery often aims at identifying a trajectory which is the closest to the presumed 'optimal' target (Fig. 1). Furthermore, there may be fewer advantages to awake surgery than commonly claimed because: (1) microelectrode recordings can be performed in GA, (2) intraoperative testing, mostly rigidity, is subjective and may be biased, e.g., towards frequently implanted trajectories, (3) the level of rigidity is constantly waning during intraoperative testing due to microlesioning effects and poorly-understood carry-over effects, making comparative rating of different trajectories difficult, (4) some patients reveal minor rigidity at surgery and rigidity cannot be reliably provoked on a constant level, (5) two trajectories may be equally efficient, (6) side-effects, such as those associated with current spread to the internal capsule can also be detected under GA, (7) the examination of speech in the surgical setting is subjective, and influenced by the severity of the OFF medication state, vigilance, and other circumstances such as dry mouth, and intraoperative testing is not sensitive with respect to daily conversation, (8) the effect of DBS on important symptoms, such as gait and akinesia, cannot be properly tested intraoperatively, and (9) overall patient cooperation in the OFF medication state is often limited. These arguments challenge the concept that awake surgery is mandatory for STN electrode implantation.

C.K.E. Moll, MD, A. Gulberti, A. Sharrott, PhD, and A.K. Engel, MD, PhD
Department of Neurophysiology and Pathophysiology, Center of Experimental Medicine, University Medical Center Hamburg-Eppendorf, Martinistrasse 52, 20246 Hamburg, Germany

S. Payer, MD, J. Köppen, MD, M. Westphal, MD, and W. Hamel, MD (✉)
Klinik für Neurochirurgie, Universitätsklinikum Hamburg-Eppendorf, Martinistrasse 52, 20246 Hamburg, Germany
e-mail: whamel@uke.uni-hamburg.de; whamel@uke.de

S. Zittel, MD, K. Boelmans, MD, C. Gerloff, MD, and C. Buhmann, MD
Department of Neurology, University Medical Center Hamburg-Eppendorf, Martinistrasse 52, 20246 Hamburg, Germany

C. Oehlwein, MD
Praxis für Neurologie und Psychiatrie, Lasurstrasse 27, 07551 Gera, Germany

G. Nikkhah and M. Pinsker (eds.), *Stereotactic and Functional Neurosurgery*, Acta Neurochirurgica Supplement, Vol. 117,
DOI 10.1007/978-3-7091-1482-7_4,

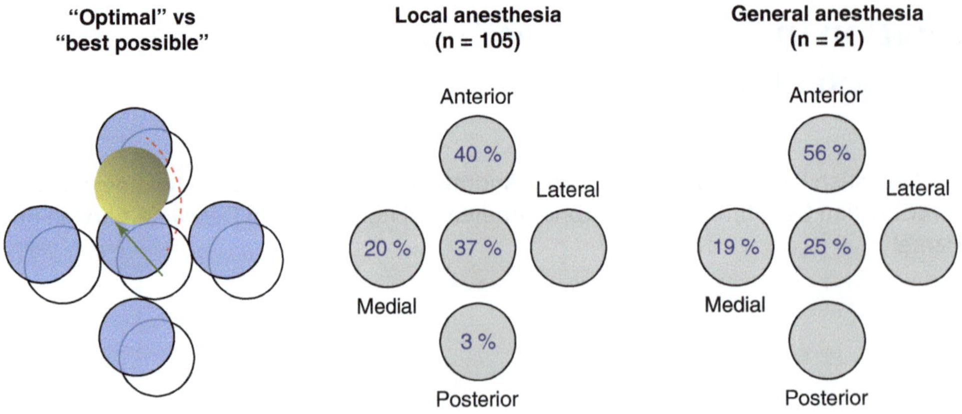

Fig. 1 The 'optimal' target (*yellow*) which is hypothesized in the *left panel* may not be exactly covered by a multielectrode approach. During surgical planning standard coordinates (*empty dots*) are modified in an attempt to get closer to the 'optimal target' (*green arrow*). Subsequently, two trajectories, i.e., central and anterior (*blue dots* connected by *red line*), may touch but still not be congruent with the hypothetical 'optimal target.' Clinical testing may reveal trajectories which are equally effective, possibly because their distance from the 'optimal' target is similar. The *middle* and *right panel* indicate the frequency with which the different trajectories were chosen for permanent electrode implantation in GA and in the awake state

Table 1 Demographic data of patients operated in general anesthesia

Patient	Sex	Age	Hx	H&Y	Reason for GA
#1	F	70	30	4	Refused LA (previous procedure in LA had to be interrupted) + gastroesophageal reflux
#2	F	52	29	4	Bedridden + anxiety + limited cooperation
#3	F	71	11	4	Painful OFF-dystonia with chest and laryngeal symptoms + claustrophobia + anxiety + age
#4	M	61	15	3	Severe OFF + not cooperative (reintubation)
#5	M	65	15	3	Patient felt unable to cope with awake surgery and GA was requested
#6	M	71	20	3	Respitatory problems b/o cervical 'dystonia' and difficult positioning + hallucinations preop (reintubation)
#7	M	53	4	3	Patient breaks fixation pins with a sudden movement during wake-up from GA (reintubation)
#8	F	69	13	4	GA requested by patient, only moderate rigidity (insufficient for intraoperative testing)
#9	M	58	15	4	Limited cooperation, restlessness
#10	M	69	20	3	Respiratory distress
#11	M	62	10	2	Limited cooperation and respiratory depression from low doses of remifentanyl (reintubation)

The reasons leading to surgery in general anaesthesia are listed
Hx time from diagnosis of Parkinson's disease until surgery, *H&Y* Hoehn and Yahr stage

In addition, the feasibility of STN stimulation in GA with an outcome similar to awake surgery has been demonstrated in several studies [1, 3–6, 8–12]. Up to now, there is no level I or level A evidence according to 'evidence-based medicine' ('EBM'), and it is unlikely to be obtained in the future.

Patients and Methods

From July 2005 to August 2009, in 11 consecutive patients suffering from advanced PD (out of 85 PD patients that were operated in our hospital during this period), STN electrodes were implanted in GA (intravenous propofol, 3–9 mg/kg/h, and remifentanil, 0.05–0.3 μg/kg/min). Demographic data and the reason for choosing general anaesthesia are summarized in Table 1. Surgery was performed as reported previously [2, 7]. In brief, simultaneous microelectrode recordings (impedances, 0.3–0.8 MΩ at 1,000 Hz) were obtained from up to five parallel tracks using four outer electrodes arranged in a concentric array around a central track aiming at the target (Ben's gun configuration; interelectrode distance 2 mm; MicroGuide, Alpha-Omega, Nazareth, Israel). Monopolar test-stimulation (60 μs; 130 Hz) was performed after reduction of propofol and remifentanil using the uninsulated macrotip of the electrode (cathodal, impedance < 1 kΩ) against the respective guide tube (anodal), with a focus on stimulation-induced limb (in particular finger) movements as well as thorough polygraphic electromyography (EMG) monitoring from flexor and extensor muscles of the upper and lower extremities. Test-stimulation was also performed with low frequencies (2–6 Hz, 100 μs) in order to provoke rhythmic muscle contractions which, however, were inconsistently observed. Thorough postoperative test-stimulation of each contact of both electrodes (model

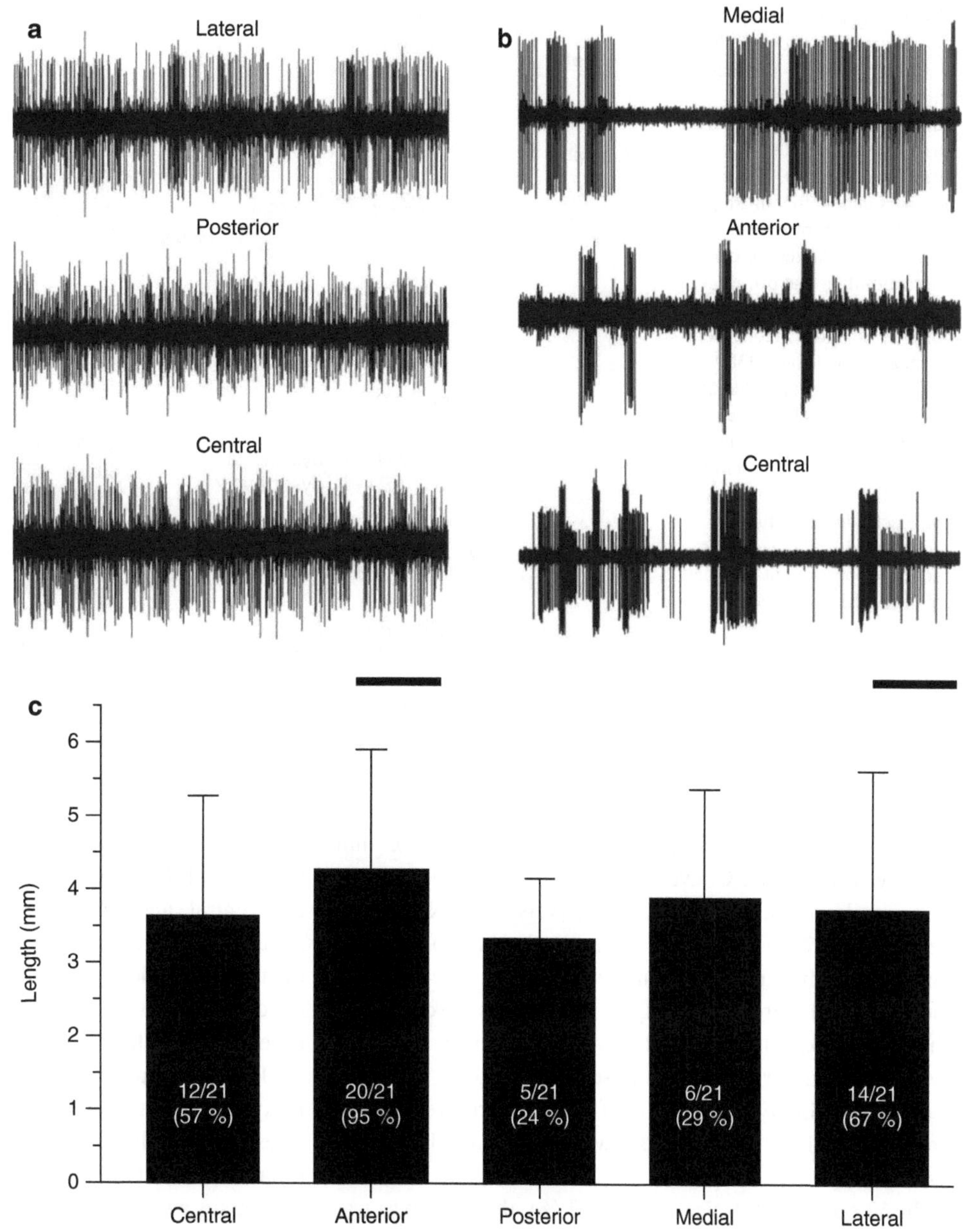

Fig. 2 Raw traces depicting typical microelectrode recording patterns during STN surgery in the awake state and in GA. **a** In the awake state, STN activity is characterized by tonic irregular firing and oscillatory bursting in the beta- or tremor-frequency range. Scale bar, 1 s. **b** The discharge pattern of STN cells in GA (patient #3, right hemisphere) clearly differs from the awake condition. Note the long interburst intervals between the unusually long group discharges, which also lead to a better recognition of neighbouring STN units. **c** Synoptic summary of the average length of STN neuronal activity recorded from different trajectories. The numbers indicate the frequency with which STN activity could be recorded from a given trajectory. Note that the anterior track traversed the STN in 95 % of all cases

DBS 3389, Medtronic Inc., Minneapolis, MN, USA) was performed following levodopa withdrawal, in order to assess the effects of stimulation on rigidity, speech, and possible side-effects resulting from current spread to the internal capsule and other neighbouring structures.

Results

In awake patients undergoing STN surgery, the penetration of the fiber capsule dorsal to the nucleus is associated with a strong increase in background activity. We found that this microphysiological hallmark is not discernible in microelectrode recordings under GA (with the propofol doses used). Nonetheless, the STN could clearly be delineated by a characteristic bursting discharge pattern which clearly differed from the prototypical low threshold spike bursts that dominated thalamic activity under GA, and which contrasted with the tonic high-frequency activity of neurons recorded from the subjacent substantia nigra, pars reticulata. In contrast to both the tonic irregular activity and oscillatory bursting which are frequently observed in the sensorimotor STN territory of awake PD patients (Fig. 2a), the bursts observed under GA often had a long duration consisting of >10 spikes, and were interspersed with long interburst intervals of absolute quiescence (Fig. 2b). In general, higher concentrations of propofol/remifentanil led to an increase of these silent

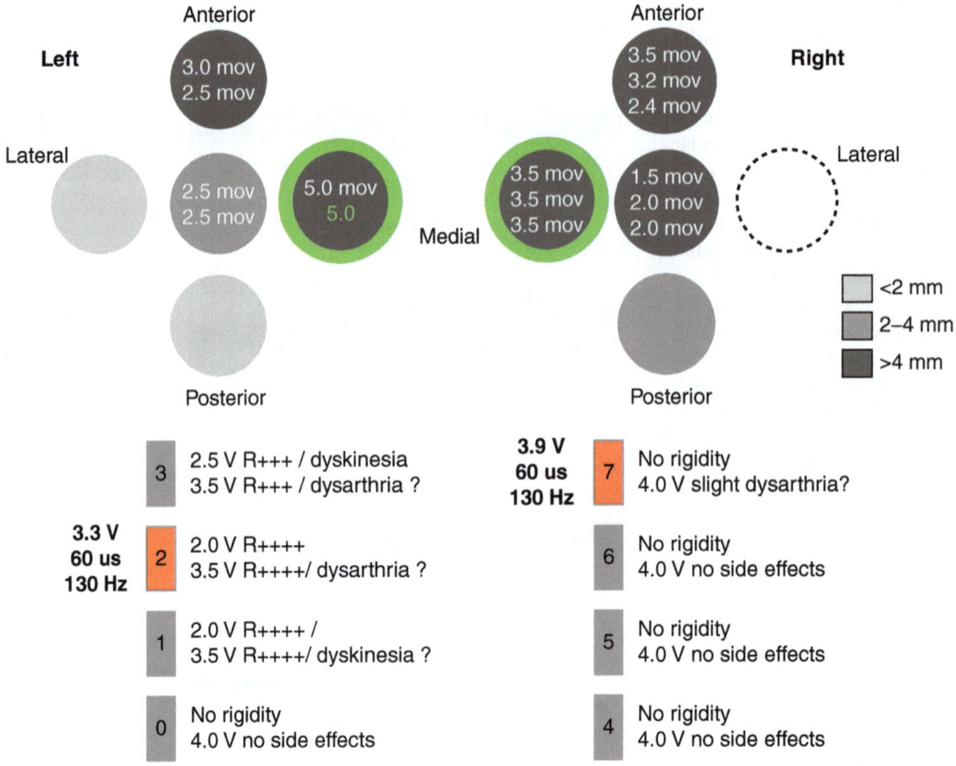

Fig. 3 The *upper panel* depicts the results from microelectrode recordings and test-stimulation in patient #1. The length of microelectrode recordings from the STN are indicated by different *grey* tones. The *white* numbers denote the threshold (mA) for motor responses (mov) elicited in the fingers or hand by microstimulation at different levels along the trajectory. *Green* numbers, no side-effects. Both permanent Medtronic 3389 electrodes were implanted along the medial tracks (*green circles*), which was in line with a third ventricle width of only 3 mm. *Below*, the results of postoperative electrode evaluation are summarized, and the contacts chosen for permanent stimulation are indicated in *orange*

interburst intervals, and reduced the overall level of unit activity in the STN. Conversely, when propofol concentration was lowered, the interburst intervals of STN neurons became progressively shorter, ultimately leading to the well-known tonic irregular firing in these cells, together with an increase in background activity as the patients woke up (not shown). As expected, and in line with the absence of clinical symptoms, tremor cells or beta oscillatory activity were not recorded in GA. Further details of the single cell recordings under GA will be published elsewhere (Moll et al., unpublished data).

In 57 out of 105 trajectories (54.2 %), the STN was traversed, as evidenced by the characteristic single-cell discharges. The average length of sampled STN activity was 3.9 ± 1.6 mm (±SD; range, 1–6.5 mm). Figure 2c provides an overview of the incidence of STN activity on individual tracks and their respective lengths.

Similarly to patients operated in the awake state, the length of sampled STN activity may be used to map the extent of the nucleus. For example, in patient #1, long segments of STN activity were encountered on the medial and anterior microelectrode tracks, which was in accordance with a width of the third ventricle of only 3 mm (Fig. 3). During test-stimulation with the central and anterior microelectrodes we found a relatively low threshold for the induction of finger and hand movements, which prompted us to implant the macroelectrodes through the medial trajectories in both hemispheres (Fig. 3). In the other ten patients reported here, only one electrode was implanted along the medial trajectory. All the remaining electrodes were implanted along the central and anterior trajectories (Table 2). In most instances, the trajectories that were actually chosen for permanent electrode implantation had revealed the highest incidence of STN single-cell recordings, except for the lateral trajectory, which traversed the STN in 67 % of all targeted nuclei but was precluded from implantation due to its proximity to the internal capsule, as evidenced by the lowest thresholds for elicitation of tonic muscle contractions of contralateral muscles. Notably, the patterns of implantation in GA versus awake surgery were similar (Fig. 1).

None of the patients displayed current spread (monopolar stimulation with at least 4.0 V, 60 μs, 130 Hz) to the corticospinal tract resulting in contraction of the face or extremities during postoperative evaluation of each contact. As shown in Fig. 3 for patient #1, the improvement of rigidity was rated, and detailed attention was given to side-effects, in particular dysarthria. In all patients, the contacts appearing most effective could be used for permanent DBS. This resulted in alleviated non-axial motor symptoms, as evidenced by improved scores in the motor subsection of the Unified Parkinson's Disease Rating Scale (UPDRS III) and a reduction of the levodopa equivalent daily dose (LEDD, summarized in Table 2; average preoperative LEDD 1,300 mg).

Bipolar stimulation in patient #3 was necessary in order to minimize unwanted effects on speech. In the other patients,

Table 2 Summary of pre- and postoperative clinical data

Patient	Mattis preop	UPDRS III Off	Dopa test	UPDRS III % improv	LEDD % reduct	f/u	Traj (L/R)	Stim left (contact / V)	Stim right (contact / V)
#1	ND[a]	58	38	ND	37	2	M / M	2+3– / 3.9	6– / 3.3
#2	140	78	54	77	47	6	A / A	2–3– / 3.3	6–7– / 3.3
#3	140	46	59	63	80	1	C / M	6–7+ / 3.4	2–1+ / 3.6
#4	139	37	41	73	65	3.5	A / A	1–2– / 3.0	5–6– / 2.7
#5	142	49	41	76	16	2.0	C / C	2– / 4.1	6– / 3.6
#6	141	34	44	62	12	4.0	A / A	1–2– / 3.0	5–6– / 3.0
#7	144	31	29[b]	42	55	3.5	A / A	3– / 3.0[d]	7– / 3.0[d]
#8	142	26	39	27	76	0.5	A / A	2– / 1.8	6– / 1.8
#9	143	21	38	19	69	1	C / A	1–2– / 3.0	9–10– / 3.0
#10	142	50	32	64	16	2	A / –[c]	1–2– / 3.0	*4–5–6– / 3.5*[e]
#11	140	23	43	70	12	2	C / A	1–2– / 3.2	5–6– / 3.0
Mean	*141*	*41*	*41*	*57*	*45*	*2.5*			

Dopa test levodopa testing, i.e., preoperative improvement of the UPDRS III scale (in percent) in the ON medication state compared to the OFF state, *UPDRS III % improv* postoperative improvement in the stimulation ON/medication ON condition at follow-up compared to preoperative OFF state, *LEDD reduct* percentage reduction in levodopa equivalence daily dose at follow-up, *f/u* follow-up in years, *Traj L/R* trajectories chosen for permanent electrode implantation, *C* central, *M* medial, *A* anterior, *Stim* stimulation parameter at follow-up for the left and right electrode; where the anode is not indicated monopolar stimulation was performed; in several patients more than one contact served as cathode; all contacts were stimulated with 60 μs and 130 Hz, except in patient #7

[a] In patient #1, the Mattis Dementia Rating Scale score had not been obtained; the Mini-Mental Status score was 27 (out of 30)

[b] Worst OFF was not attained and severe bilateral, levodopa non-responsive tremor was present

[c] Implantation of a second STN electrode for bilateral stimulation after patient had received unilateral STN stimulation more than 12 years ago

[d] Stimulation was performed with 150 Hz) and patient #10

[e] Pulse width of the previously implanted electrode was 90 μs

chronic DBS did not impair speech by an extent that had prevented monopolar stimulation. Bicathodic stimulation in several patients also indicated that chronic stimulation was not limited by intolerable side-effects. The higher stimulation frequency chosen in one of the patients (patient #7) led to a better suppression of resting tremor.

We observed no surgical complications (hemorrhage or postoperative infection). Two patients developed a transient state of confusion after the operation. One patient developed a postoperative manic phase treated by lowering stimulation parameters, and clozapine was continued. One postoperative pneumonia required treatment with antibiotics. Two patients developed postoperative incontinentia, which had improved at follow-up visits.

Discussion

The data from our retrospective, single-center, non-controlled, and non-randomized study suggests that STN surgery in GA can be performed in a safe manner resulting in improved motor symptoms and reduced LEDD. We present our implantation technique, which is based on a combination of intraoperative microelectrode recordings and test-stimulation. The STN could clearly be delineated by intraoperative microrecordings, although the typical increase in background noise was not observed, which has also been reported by Hertel et al. [4]. The corticospinal tract can be determined and avoided by intraoperative test-stimulation, as demonstrated in one of our patients (Fig. 3). Following surgery, current spread to the corticospinal tract using conventional stimulation parameters and above was not observed in any of the patients. In addition, there were no side-effects which could be attributed to surgery in GA. It seems rather unlikely that the side-effects actually observed would have been prevented by surgery in the awake state (e.g., postoperative mania was not due to ventromedial electrode implantation).

One may argue that in the awake state motor symptoms had improved even further, and LEDD reduction had been higher. Nevertheless, the improvements we have observed are in the range of what can be expected for a common PD patient cohort. In addition, most of the patients were severely affected and, indeed, they required surgery in GA.

In particular, from a technical viewpoint less clinical improvement following STN surgery in GA can be regarded as unlikely, since the trajectories selected for permanent electrode implantation compared well to patients operated in the awake state. When using the ‘Ben’s gun’ approach, the choice of the trajectory is practically *the only* relevant variable for the site of permanent electrode position, since electrode depth can be equalized postoperatively by the choice of appropriate contacts. The other factor determining the location of the electrode, i.e., stereotactic planning, is not influenced by the mode of anaesthesia.

Our data are in agreement with an elaborate study in which 54 patients were assigned at random to surgery in the awake state ($n=24$) or GA ($n=30$) [5]. Although, the absolute values were slightly in favour of awake surgery, they detected no statistically significant difference between awake surgery and GA with regard to the stimulation parameters used and all the scores assessed, i.e., Hoehn & Yahr stage, UPDRS II, III, and IV, and LEDD reduction [5]. In two smaller studies, slight differences in favor of awake surgery have been reported [6, 12]. Furthermore, cognitive decline has been reported in one study in which GA was induced with desflurane [1].

Although many would ask for a randomized controlled trial (RCT) to ultimately clear this issue, it should be kept in mind that even a meta-analysis of a number of prospective, multicenter RCTs may eventually not solve some of the well-known challenges of so-called ‘evidence-based medicine.’ That is: (1) RCTs tend to confirm what sound and convincing studies had suggested, i.e., the equivalence of awake surgery and GA has been demonstrated in the study of Lefaucheur et al. [5], (2) even if we assume that patients operated in the awake state fare (slightly) better, the applicability of such data to an individual patient, possibly not even meeting the inclusion criteria of the RCT, is limited, and (3) data from multicentric RCT may be of value for a general assessment of STN surgery in GA but cannot necessarily be transferred to different centers, since details of the intraoperative approach have an important impact on the success of the procedure (e.g., technique of microelectrode recordings and test-stimulation, mode of anaesthesia, i.e., intravenous vs inhalational).

In conjunction with the studies already available, careful analysis of single-center data (in full awareness of the methodological limitations, i.e., retrospective, non-controlled, non-randomized) may already provide excellent information to advise patients requesting or requiring STN surgery in GA. Our study was not intended to clear the way for STN surgery in GA on a routine basis. There are no obvious advantages of STN surgery in GA, except for patient comfort and, under certain circumstances, patient safety. Whenever the decision is made, possible risks associated with prolonged general anaesthesia, in particular in Parkinson’s disease, have also to be considered.

This study does not address differential costs associated with both approaches. STN stimulation performed in general anaesthesia may be more profitable (e.g., implantation of electrodes and stimulator within the same session) or may result in higher expenses (e.g., analgetics and sedatives).

Conflict of Interest The authors have occasionally been reimbursed for travel expenses and received honoraria from Medtronic Inc. for speaking at meetings.

References

1. Chen SY, Tsai ST, Lin SH, Chen TY, Hung HY, Lee CW, Wang WH, Chen SP, Lin SZ (2011) Subthalamic deep brain stimulation in Parkinson's disease under different anesthetic modalities: a comparative cohort study. Stereotact Funct Neurosurg 89:372–380
2. Hamel W, Fietzek U, Morsnowski A, Schrader B, Herzog J, Weinert D, Pfister G, Muller D, Volkmann J, Deuschl G, Mehdorn HM (2003) Deep brain stimulation of the subthalamic nucleus in Parkinson's disease: evaluation of active electrode contacts. J Neurol Neurosurg Psychiatry 74:1036–1046
3. Harries AM, Kausar J, Roberts SA, Mocroft AP, Hodson JA, Pall HS, Mitchell RD (2011) Deep brain stimulation of the subthalamic nucleus for advanced Parkinson disease using general anesthesia: long-term results. J Neurosurg 116:107–113
4. Hertel F, Zuchner M, Weimar I, Gemmar P, Noll B, Bettag M, Decker C (2006) Implantation of electrodes for deep brain stimulation of the subthalamic nucleus in advanced Parkinson's disease with the aid of intraoperative microrecording under general anesthesia. Neurosurgery 59:E1138; discussion E1138
5. Lefaucheur JP, Gurruchaga JM, Pollin B, von Raison F, Mohsen N, Shin M, Menard-Lefaucheur I, Oshino S, Kishima H, Fenelon G, Remy P, Cesaro P, Gabriel I, Brugieres P, Keravel Y, Nguyen JP (2008) Outcome of bilateral subthalamic nucleus stimulation in the treatment of Parkinson's disease: correlation with intra-operative multi-unit recordings but not with the type of anaesthesia. Eur Neurol 60:186–199
6. Maltete D, Navarro S, Welter ML, Roche S, Bonnet AM, Houeto JL, Mesnage V, Pidoux B, Dormont D, Cornu P, Agid Y (2004) Subthalamic stimulation in Parkinson disease: with or without anesthesia? Arch Neurol 61:390–392
7. Moll CK, Sharott A, Hamel W, Munchau A, Buhmann C, Hidding U, Zittel S, Westphal M, Muller D, Engel AK (2009) Waking up the brain: a case study of stimulation-induced wakeful unawareness during anaesthesia. Prog Brain Res 177:125–145
8. Nakajima T, Zrinzo L, Foltynie T, Olmos IA, Taylor C, Hariz MI, Limousin P (2011) MRI-guided subthalamic nucleus deep brain stimulation without microelectrode recording: can we dispense with surgery under local anaesthesia? Stereotact Funct Neurosurg 89:318–325
9. Patel NK, Plaha P, Gill SS (2007) Magnetic resonance imaging-directed method for functional neurosurgery using implantable guide tubes. Neurosurgery 61:358–365; discussion 365–356
10. Starr PA, Martin AJ, Ostrem JL, Talke P, Levesque N, Larson PS (2010) Subthalamic nucleus deep brain stimulator placement using high-field interventional magnetic resonance imaging and a skull-mounted aiming device: technique and application accuracy. J Neurosurg 112:479–490
11. Sutcliffe AJ, Mitchell RD, Gan YC, Mocroft AP, Nightingale P (2011) General anaesthesia for deep brain stimulator electrode insertion in Parkinson's disease. Acta Neurochir (Wien) 153:621–627
12. Yamada K, Goto S, Kuratsu J, Matsuzaki K, Tamura T, Nagahiro S, Murase N, Shimazu H, Kaji R (2007) Stereotactic surgery for subthalamic nucleus stimulation under general anesthesia: a retrospective evaluation of Japanese patients with Parkinson's disease. Parkinsonism Relat Disord 13:101–107

The Impact of Multichannel Microelectrode Recording (MER) in Deep Brain Stimulation of the Basal Ganglia

Thomas M. Kinfe and Jan Vesper

Abstract Deep brain stimulation (DBS) of the basal ganglia (Ncl. subthalamicus, Ncl. ventralis intermedius thalami, globus pallidus internus) has become an evidence-based and well-established treatment option in otherwise refractory movement disorders. The Ncl. subthalamicus (STN) is the target of choice in Parkinson's disease.

However, a considerable discussion is currently ongoing with regard to the necessity for micro-electrode recording (MER) in DBS surgery.

The present review provides an overview on deep brain stimulation and (MER) of the STN in patients with Parkinson's disease. Detailed description is given concerning the multichannel MER systems nowadays available for DBS of the basal ganglia, especially of the STN, as a useful tool for target refinement. Furthermore, an overview is given of the historical aspects, spatial mapping of the STN by MER, and its impact for accuracy and precision in current functional stereotactic neurosurgery.

The pros concerning target refinement by MER means on the one hand, and cons including increased bleeding risk, increased operation time, local or general anesthesia, and single versus multichannel microelectrode recording are discussed in detail. Finally, the authors favor the use of MER with intraoperative testing combined with imaging to achieve a more precise electrode placement, aiming to ameliorate clinical outcome in therapy-resistant movement disorders.

Keywords Deep brain stimulation • Basal ganglia • Microelectrode recording • Movement disorders

T.M. Kinfe, MD (✉) and J. Vesper, MD, PhD
Center of Neuromodulation, Department of Neurosurgery, Heinrich-Heine University Hospital,
Moorenstrasse 5, Düsseldorf 40225, Germany
e-mail: thomas.kinfe@med.uni-duesseldorf.de

History

The internal globus pallidus (GPi) and the ventrolateral thalamus (Vim) are well-established targets in the treatment of movement disorders. With the introduction of the modern era of deep brain stimulation, pathophysiological superordinate subthalamic nucleus (STN) came into focus as a proposed target in Parkinson's disease (PD). Functional procedures were performed in the subthalamic area in the 1960s [5].

Struppler, who first reported microphysiological recordings in the subthalamic area, observed marked tremor reduction and used neurolesions to implant microelectrode devices. The efficacy of subthalamotomy was attributed to the fact that the pallidofugal and dentatothalamic pathways were altered by the employed microelectrode devices [66]. The earlier performed ablative procedure led to distortion of the fields of Forel and the zona incerta within the realm of the radiation prelemniscalis, whereas involvement of the STN caused severe hemiballism [14].

Bergmann et al. described that lesioning of the STN in 1-methyl-4-phenyl-1,2,3,6-tetrahydropyridin-treated primates reduced Parkinsonian symptoms without inducing hemiballism [10]. This finding was confirmed by Benabid et al. in humans, which again drew attention to the STN in functional neurosurgery and contributed to the superior denotation of the STN in the treatment of advanced PD [8, 57].

Introduction

Dopaminergic degeneration in the substantia nigra reflects the common morphological earmark in advanced Parkinson's disease (PD), which leads to dopamine deficiency in the striatum via nigrostriatal projections. There is evidence that in PD or essential tremor (ET), this nigrostriatal degeneration induces neuronal activity changes in different brain structures that enclose the sensorimotor cortex and the subcortical areas,

G. Nikkhah and M. Pinsker (eds.), *Stereotactic and Functional Neurosurgery*, Acta Neurochirurgica Supplement, Vol. 117,
DOI 10.1007/978-3-7091-1482-7_5,

namely the ventrolateral thalamus and the basal ganglia (striatum, internal/external globus pallidus, subthalamic nucleus). In particular, these subcortical structures were not amenable to electrophysiological mapping at demanding intervals, using electrophysiologically-based target refinement [17, 72].

The pathophysiological mechanisms have been poorly understood in the past two decades, since the introduction of deep brain stimulation (DBS) as a treatment modality for movement disorders, notably tremor symptoms, provided new insight into our comprehension of the genesis of movement disorders [6, 44, 58, 60].

The use of microelectrode recording (MER) prior to implantation of the final DBS electrodes in awake patients is now well-established. Target refinement can be performed safely and accurately using electrophysiological data acquisition. Single-cell recording studies can also be analyzed and correlated to accessory electrophysiological data such as muscle or cortical activity, which provides new insight into the pathophysiological mechanism. Furthermore, pathological firing patterns can have direct therapeutic implications.

Experimental animal models for PD such as 1-methyl-4-phenyl-1,2,3,6-tetrahydropyridin treatment in primates revealed tremor-associated firing patterns in the subthalamic nucleus (STN) and the internal globus pallidus (GPi) [11, 71]. Introduced in the 1960s, neurophysiological mapping may provide insight into the poorly understood pathophysiology of several movement disorders.

Intraoperative MER of the basal ganglia, the STN in particular, along the trajectory to a target is recommended to ensure three-dimensional disbandment of the proposed target area. Therefore, the proposed target areas can be distinguished by their characteristic discharge patterns, namely the thalamus, the pallidum, the STN, and the substantia nigra.

Hyperactivity of the STN and the GPi in patients with PD reveals characteristic irregular discharge patterns, so-called "bursts" [13, 20, 22, 24, 32, 37]. MER undoubtedly contributes to our understanding of the functional organization of the basal ganglia, allowing spatial assignment of the functional target, e.g., the STN. Analysis of the spontaneous neuronal activity along the trajectory is necessary for STN identification. The characteristic discharge patterns helps distinguish neuronal formations (according to the underlying disorder in the STN, GPi, or Vim), particularly the nucleus reticularis of the thalamus and its anterior border, the superior and inferior border of the STN, and the substantia nigra (Snr). Irregular high-frequency discharge patterns can be found in advanced PD in the STN and the GPi. According to frequency and amplitude, graphic and statistical debriefing can be performed to differentiate the proposed target from nearby subcortical structures. The precision and accuracy of the electrode placement impact the success of the functional procedure. MER of neuronal activity reflects a fundamental orientation facility prior to target refinement. Four-contact macroelectrodes are typically used for permanent stimulation; for that reason, guidance along the trajectory, during which characteristic discharges can be detected, may be helpful to achieve the most beneficial high-frequency stimulation along this distance. Until now, there has been no evidence of a correlation between the amplitude of the firing patterns and clinical effect [16, 25, 32, 41, 48, 55, 63, 70].

Anesthesia

Stereotactic-guided implantation of DBS electrodes for the treatment of movement disorders, for advanced PD in particular, is performed by standardized surgical procedure means. This, definitely, can differ among neurosurgical centers. Controversy exists with regard to not only the need for MER but also whether the surgical procedure should be performed under local or general anesthesia. There are some considerations against general anesthesia, including the following: (1) interpretation of the assessed mapping is hindered, (2) identification of the sensorimotor portion of the target is impossible or limited, which holds true for intraoperative testing via macrostimulation, aiming to determine threshold values of beneficial stimulation-induced side-effects, (3) surgery-related complications may be disguised, and (4) use of the awake functional procedure obtains better results pertaining to clinical outcome [23, 35, 36, 42, 45, 50, 56, 63, 68].

In contrast, general anesthesia may be helpful for patients in whom surgery otherwise could not be performed, PD patients with severe off state, patients with dystonia and a distinct phasic component, and patients in whom aspiration must be avoided. In all of these conditions, the use of MER is possible, but one should cautiously interpret the electrophysiological findings.

Both advantages and disadvantages can be compensated by the use of an analogosedative regime. Patients can be guided in a sedative manner for the first surgical steps (frame fixation, planning, and burr-hole placement) with propofol (Disoprivan®) and a short-lasting analgesic such as remifentanil (Ultiva®). Additionally, especially in PD patients, the off period until recording can be shortened or reduced with continuous apomorphine administration using an apomorphine pump, which is fast exhalable and does not influence the motor responsiveness. One has to consider that patient alertness or drug application (e.g., hypnotic or sedative) may influence the neuronal spontaneous firing patterns of subcortical structures, as evidenced by blurred recordings [21, 28, 39, 46, 52–54]. This contortion is notable in microrecordings under general anesthesia (e.g., patients with dystonia).

Both the frequency/pattern of neuronal activity and the background noise may make valuable contributions to differentiation of the proposed target area. The background activity can be seen proportional to the cell density in a defined area, and is independent from impacts discussed above. For instance, background activity is very low in the

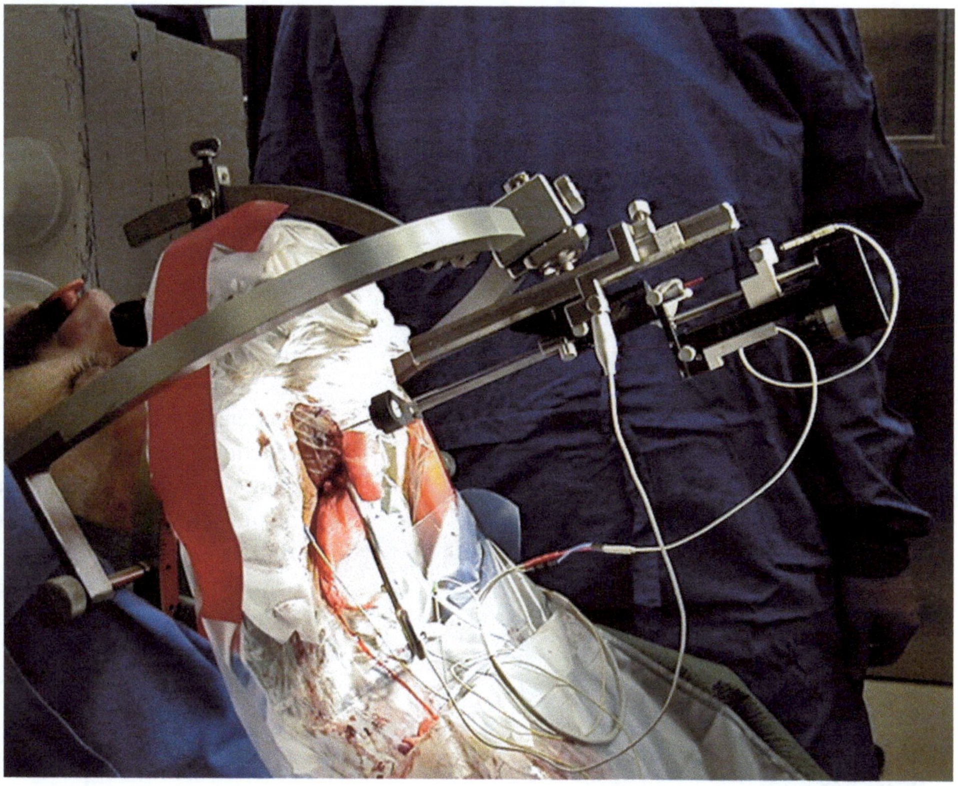

Fig. 1 Combined micro/macroelectrode (Inomed, Teningen, Germany) in situ with manual microdrive (Medtronic, Minneapolis, MN, USA)

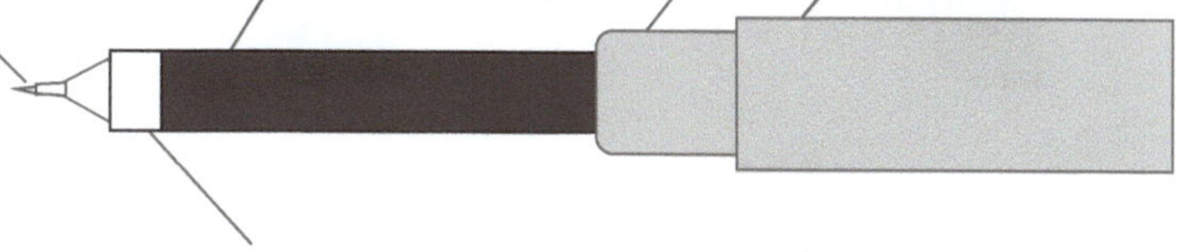

Fig. 2 Combined micro/macroelectrode (Inomed, Teningen, Germany)

zona incerta, but increases upon entry to the STN because of the cellular density of the STN [1, 43, 47, 71].

Technique

Microelectrodes are available with platinum–iridium and wolfram-tip. The small micro-tip surface and size allow for high outlet impedance of 0.5–1.5 MΩ. Repetitive microstimulation is possible, but after several stimulations, it must be replaced because of decreased impedance (Fig. 1).

The multichannel MER requires the use of a sufficient electrode sheath and amplifier/recording system. MER can be performed as a parallel multi-channel recording or a sequential single-channel recording, each of which has specific advantages and disadvantages, and neither of which has been proven superior over the other. Sequential one-channel recording requires greater surgical experience, since addition trajectory is necessary in cases of unsatisfactory clinical response and recording. The proposed targets can be demarcated from nearby structures; moreover, typical neuronal discharges of different frequencies and rhythmicities of tremor-correlated anatomical structures can be detected.

The use of parallel multichannel recording enables parallel testing of different trajectories along the z-axis to allow spatial orientation in the case of stimulation-induced side-effects. The placement of the electrodes can be verified using intraoperative testing combined with neurological examination, since nearly 40 % of the performed DBS implantations require electrode location correction [12, 16, 19, 24, 29, 32, 37, 56, 62, 64, 73]. For that purpose, the use of a combined micro/macroelectrode appears appropriate to achieve a close-mesh spatial correlation between the micro-recording and the test stimulation (Fig. 2).

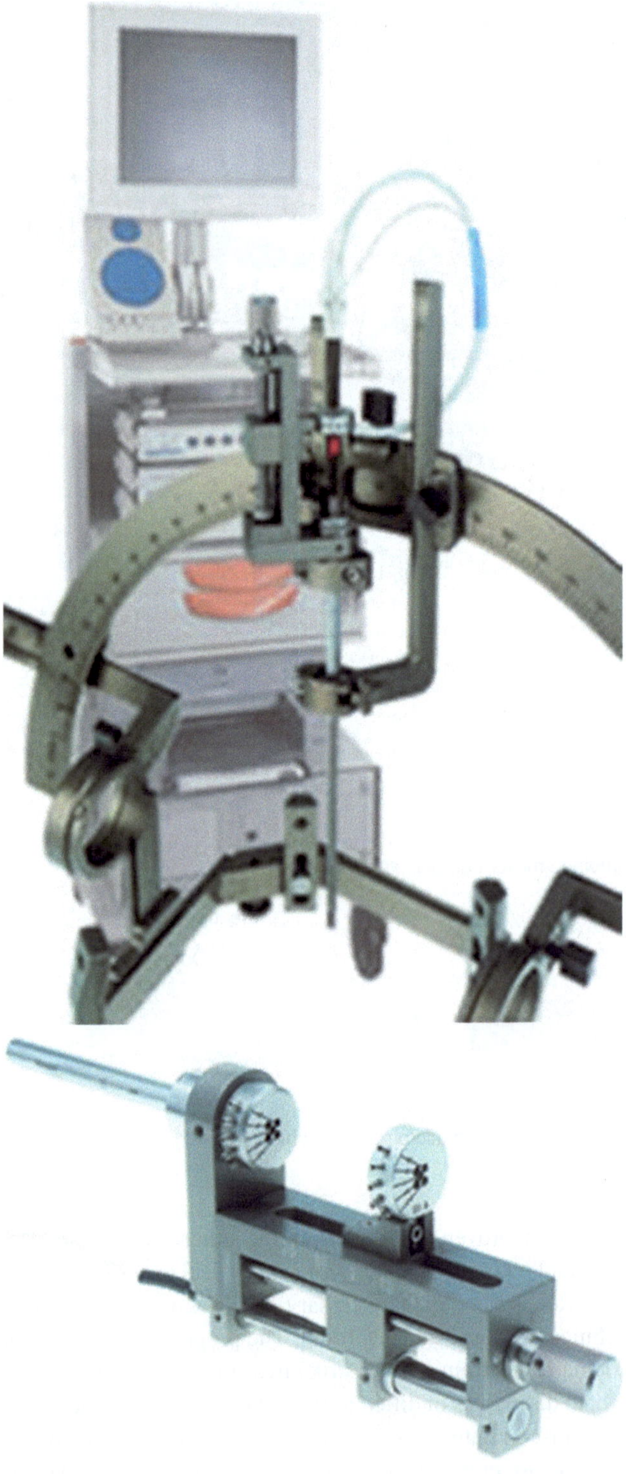

Fig. 3 The microelectrode recording system (Inomed, Teningen, Germany), a microdrive with five parallel trajectories

Micro- and Macroelectrodes

The scope of the micro/macroelectrode involves neurophysiologically refining the proposed target area. Various manual and automatic recording microdrive systems are available. The outer diameter of the electrode is reduced to 0.5–0.8 mm, whereas the tip gauges are 2–4 μm; therefore, it is suitable for single-cell recording.

The distance between the micro- and macroelectrode can vary; for instance, the Inomed micro- and macroelectrode tip is fixed and has a length of 15 mm, while FHC provides a flexible microelectrode tip that can be driven out to 10 mm below the macroelectrode. Maximum spike amplitude is possible because of the low capacity of the electrode measurement. The 'Ben's gun' system, which facilitates the insertion of up to five microelectrodes (Fig. 3), is required for multichannel recording. This accessible microdrive system enables insertion of up to five microelectrodes during functional surgery; otherwise, the functional procedure can start with fewer electrodes if necessary. The annulment of 50 μm allows the functional surgeon an exact electrode localization, and is driven in half-millimeter pitches. An optional sensor transfers the electrode position to the MER recording system with parallel visualization. Using this tool, precise and fast intervention and clinico-neurological appraisal of the stimulation effects on the target point are endorsed.

Technical Considerations

The target refinement in DBS remains controversial with regard to different recommended surgical protocols of clinical testing as well as neuroimaging modalities using image-fusion and neurophysiological techniques [2, 26, 27, 31, 51, 65]. Intraoperative fusion of images from different imaging modalities for target verification reflects a pivotal step for accurate target refinement; in contrast, relying on one MR sequence for target verification leads to misplacements. For indirect targeting, anatomical landmarks such as the anterior and posterior commissura and other midline-related structures are required. For delineation of the midline structures, the use of ventriculography (although not currently), computed tomography, or MR scans is suitable, multiple findings of which can be fused to leverage the advantages of each modality [7, 18, 34, 67, 73]. The essential components of this functional procedure include path-planning (trajectory) and the distance in which MER can be performed. The trajectory must be chosen carefully, to avoid contact with the ventricular wall and blood vessels between the cortical surface and the target, at an angle that contributes to the anatomical compass of the proposed target.

The efficacy of MER can be increased with parallel insertion of five microelectrodes with an interspace of 2 mm. In the case of anatomical variation (subcortical atrophy, atypical blood vessel course, anomalies), the number of inserted microelectrodes must be reduced to avoid hemorrhagic complications. The probing of the target area reflects for each electrode a certain depth profile, allowing the generation of a reliable electrophysiological mapping of targeted brain structures with different activity patterns [4]. Among five microelectrode-recordings, the one that strains the target at the longest distance and possesses the highest rate of neuronal discharge patterns must be chosen. In the next step, test stimulation can be performed that encompasses the functional mapping of the proposed target.

Maximal suppression of motor symptoms by test stimulation means without the induction of side-effects is ideal. Afterward, the four-contact permanent electrode is placed with its second lowest contact on the target level.

Due to the fact that the STN is a relatively small nucleus (diameter 5–6 mm) MER-guided target refinement to identify the proposed sensorimotor part of the STN that encompass its anterolateral portion, MER sometimes can be crucial [4].

MER generally starts 10 mm above the estimated target. The nucleus areas of the basal ganglia display a spontaneous firing pattern of approximately 80 Hz. Low-frequency firing neurons can also be detected in the striatum or zona incerta. In addition to the average spontaneous firing rate, the time course of the neuronal activity is an essential contributor to target refinement. Above the STN, irregular low-frequency patterns from the anterior thalamus (ncl. reticularis) can be detected, whereas non-specific patterns can be found in the zona incerta. Within the STN, stable and high-frequency irregular bursts with high amplitude appear. The time period of electrical stabilization after microelectrode insertion could last several minutes. In this time period, no or non-specific patterns can occur, so that slow forwarding with the microdrive is warranted and limits the usefulness of an electric-guided microdrive [3, 4, 15, 16, 19, 24, 32, 61, 65, 73].

According to our experience, valid and reliable data quality can be achieved using a 0.5–1.0-mm microdrive setting. Additionally, the muscle activity of the flexors/extensors of the wrist joints using surface electrodes or EMG activity above the hand motor area using bipolar needle electrodes can be recorded and correlated to the MER findings [4, 40].

The Impact of MER

A considerable debate is ongoing regarding the necessity of MER in DBS surgery. While some authors favor this technique, others report an increased bleeding risk without substantial impact for target refinement.

One criticism of the use of MER is its inconsistent interindividual reproducibility. The treated disorders also have different pathophysiological backgrounds. Furthermore, the highest rate of neuronal activity does not display the region with the best clinical stimulation effect [26, 30, 32–34, 38, 49, 65, 73].

On the other hand, the reproducibility of MER-induced intraoperative bleeding complication is very low. Binder et al. reported a bleeding rate of 3.0 %, and 0.6 % of the bleeding was related to permanent neurological deficits in a total of 481 patients with implanted electrodes. Similar data were provided by several other studies [9, 12, 59]. The authors believe that MER is generally safe and efficient, with a low complication rate in terms of MER-induced intraoperative bleeding [69]. The usefulness of electrophysiological identification of the maximal STN penetration is strongly correlated with permanent DBS electrode placement [73]. Nevertheless, according to a variety of circumstances influencing the surgical outcome, direct proof of MER usefulness is sometimes insufficient.

In earlier performed functional irreversible lesioning procedures such as pallidotomy or thalamotomy, an accurately and precise target refinement was necessary in order to avoid damage to nearby brain structures with consecutive surgical-related neurological alteration. In sense of best clinical effect, this holds true for reversible DBS electrode implantation with respect to functional and anatomical target localization.

Despite the tremendous development in neuroimaging, especially of the subcortical structure, anatomic and functional determination of the target areas by neuroimaging modalities is lacking. From that point of view, MER remains indispensable for target refinement and target mapping, and secondary MER generates a functional and spatial assessment of the target and is essential for detection of the sensorimotor region within the proposed nucleus.

Increased surgical duration with a consecutively increased complication rate is another major criticism. In our retrospective evaluated data, we investigated a total of 68 DBS implantations. Thirty-six patients who underwent MER showed median surgical duration of 199 min; in contrast, 32 patients who did not undergo MER showed median surgical duration of 201 min. One must consider that parallel multichannel MER in nearly 40 % of the cases involving trajectory other than the central trajectory (anterior, medial, lateral, posterior) should be taken into consideration [56].

Routine use of microelectrodes increases surgical material costs. Inconclusive data exist that could not demonstrate the superiority of imaging or intraoperative testing under local anesthesia compared to intraoperatively performed MER. On the other hand, none of the mentioned alternative approaches are consistent enough when performed alone; therefore, each should ideally be combined with MER for target refinement. No data are available to correlate the neuronal firing patterns with clinical outcome.

Considering our own experience and the actual published data, a distinct recommendation can be made for the use of MER in DBS.

Conflict of Interest Thomas M. Kinfe has received DBS training grant from Medtronic Inc. and training support from St. Jude Medical, Inc. Jan Vesper has been supported for travel and conference presentations from Medtronic Inc. and from St. Jude Medical, Inc.

References

1. Alexander GE, Crutcher MD (1990) Functional architecture of basal ganglia circuits: neural substrates of parallel processing [see comments]. Trends Neurosci 13:266–271
2. Alterman RL, Reiter GT, Shils J, Skolnick B, Arle JE, Lesutis M et al (1999) Targeting for thalamic deep brain stimulator implantation without computer guidance: assessment of targeting accuracy. Stereotact Funct Neurosurg 72:150–153
3. Amirnovin R, Williams ZM, Cosgrove GR, Eskandar EN (2006) Experience with microelectrode guided subthalamic nucleus deep brain stimulation. Neurosurgery 58:ONS96–ONS102
4. Amtage F, Henschel K, Schelter B, Vesper J, Timmer J, Lucking CH et al (2008) Tremor-correlated neuronal activity in the subthalamic nucleus of Parkinsonian patients. Neurosci Lett 442:195–199
5. Andy OJ, Jurko MF (1965) Alteration in Parkinson tremor during electrode insertion. Confin Neurol 26:378–381
6. Benabid AL, Benazzouz A, Hoffmann D, Limousin P, Krack P, Pollak P (1998) Long-term electrical inhibition of deep brain targets in movement disorders. Mov Disord 13(Suppl 3):119–125
7. Benabid AL, Koudsie A, Benazzouz A, Vercueil L, Fraix V, Chabardes S et al (2001) Deep brain stimulation of the corpus luysi (subthalamic nucleus) and other targets in Parkinson's disease. Extension to new indications such as dystonia and epilepsy. J Neurol 248:III37–III47
8. Benabid AL, Wallace B, Mitrofanis J, Xia R, Piallat B, Chabardes S et al (2005) A putative generalized model of the effects and mechanism of action of high frequency electrical stimulation of the central nervous system. Acta Neurol Belg 105:149–157
9. Ben Haim S, Asaad WF, Gale JT, Eskandar EN (2009) Risk factors for hemorrhage during microelectrode-guided deep brain stimulation and the introduction of an improved microelectrode design. Neurosurgery 64:754–762
10. Bergman H, Wichmann T, DeLong MR (1990) Reversal of experimental parkinsonism by lesions of the subthalamic nucleus. Science 249:1436–1438
11. Bergman H, Wichmann T, Karmon B, DeLong MR (1994) The primate subthalamic nucleus. II. Neuronal activity in the MPTP model of parkinsonism. J Neurophysiol 72:507–520
12. Binder DK, Rau GM, Starr PA (2005) Risk factors for hemorrhage during microelectrode-guided deep brain stimulator implantation for movement disorders. Neurosurgery 56:722–732
13. Burchiel KJ, Anderson VC, Favre J, Hammerstad JP (1999) Comparison of pallidal and subthalamic nucleus deep brain stimulation for advanced Parkinson's disease: results of a randomized, blinded pilot study. Neurosurgery 45:1375–1382
14. Carpenter MB, Carpenter CS (1951) Analysis of somatotropic relations of the corpus luysi in man and monkey; relation between the site of dyskinesia and distribution of lesions within the subthalamic nucleus. J Comp Neurol 95:349–370
15. Coenen VA, Gielen FL, Castro-Prado F, Abdel RA, Honey CR (2008) Noradrenergic modulation of subthalamic nucleus activity in human: metoprolol reduces spiking activity in microelectrode recordings during deep brain stimulation surgery for Parkinson's disease. Acta Neurochir (Wien) 150(8):757–762; discussion 762
16. Counelis GJ, Simuni T, Forman MS, Jaggi JL, Trojanowski JQ, Baltuch GH (2003) Bilateral subthalamic nucleus deep brain stimulation for advanced PD: correlation of intraoperative MER and postoperative MRI with neuropathological findings. Mov Disord 18:1062–1065
17. DeLong MR, Georgopoulos AP, Crutcher MD, Mitchell SJ, Richardson RT, Alexander GE (1984) Functional organization of the basal ganglia: contributions of single-cell recording studies. Ciba Found Symp 107:64–82
18. Duffner F, Schiffbauer H, Breit S, Friese S, Freudenstein D (2002) Relevance of image fusion for target point determination in functional neurosurgery. Acta Neurochir (Wien) 144:445–451
19. Falkenberg JH, McNames J, Burchiel KJ (2006) Automatic microelectrode recording analysis and visualization of the globus pallidus interna and stereotactic trajectory. Stereotact Funct Neurosurg 84:28–34
20. Favre J, Taha JM, Baumann T, Burchiel KJ (1999) Computer analysis of the tonic, phasic, and kinesthetic activity of pallidal discharges in Parkinson patients. Surg Neurol 51:665–672
21. Fedele E, Stefani A, Bassi A, Pepicelli O, Altibrandi MG, Frasca S et al (2001) Clinical and electrophysiological effects of apomorphine in Parkinson's disease patients are not paralleled by amino acid release changes: a microdialysis study. Funct Neurol 16:57–66
22. Forster A, Eljamel MS, Varma TR, Tulley M, Latimer M (1999) Audit of neurophysiological recording during movement disorder surgery. Stereotact Funct Neurosurg 72:154–156
23. Ganes T (1975) Barbiturate spindle activity in the thalamic lateral ventro-posterior nucleus and the second somato-sensory area of the cortex. Brain Res 98:473–483
24. Garonzik IM, Hua SE, Ohara S, Lenz FA (2002) Intraoperative microelectrode and semi-microelectrode recording during the physiological localization of the thalamic nucleus ventral intermediate. Mov Disord 17:S135–S144
25. Gerschlager W, Bloem BR, Alesch F, Lang W, Deecke L, Cunnington R (2001) Bilateral subthalamic nucleus stimulation does not improve prolonged P300 latencies in Parkinson's disease. J Neurol 248:285–289
26. Guridi J, Gorospe A, Ramos E, Linazasoro G, Rodriguez MC, Obeso JA (1999) Stereotactic targeting of the globus pallidus internus in Parkinson's disease: imaging versus electrophysiological mapping [see comments]. Neurosurgery 45:278–287
27. Guridi J, Rodriguez-Oroz MC, Lozano AM, Moro E, Albanese A, Nuttin B et al (2000) Targeting the basal ganglia for deep brain stimulation in Parkinson's disease. Neurology 55:S21–S28
28. Gutknecht C (2001) Parkinson therapy 2001, especially apomorphine in idiopathic Parkinson syndrome. Schweiz Rundsch Med Prax 90:1024–1034
29. Hariz M, Blomstedt P, Limousin P (2004) The myth of microelectrode recording in ensuring a precise location of the DBS electrode within the sensorimotor part of the subthalamic nucleus. Mov Disord 19:863–864
30. Hariz MI (1999) Current controversies in pallidal surgery. Adv Neurol 80:593–602
31. Hariz MI, Bergenheim AT (1990) A comparative study on ventriculographic and computerized tomography-guided determinations of brain targets in functional stereotaxis. J Neurosurg 73:565–571
32. Hariz MI, Fodstad H (1999) Do microelectrode techniques increase accuracy or decrease risks in pallidotomy and deep brain stimulation? A critical review of the literature. Stereotact Funct Neurosurg 72:157–169
33. Hariz MI, Fodstad H (2002) Deep brain stimulation in Parkinson's disease. N Engl J Med 346:452–453
34. Hirabayashi H, Hariz MI, Fagerlund M (1998) Comparison between stereotactic CT and MRI coordinates of pallidal and thalamic targets using the Laitinen noninvasive stereoadapter. Stereotact Funct Neurosurg 71:117–130
35. Kalenka A, Schwarz A (2009) Anaesthesia and Parkinson's disease: how to manage with new therapies? Curr Opin Anaesthesiol 22:419–424
36. Khatib R, Ebrahim Z, Rezai A, Cata JP, Boulis NM, John DD et al (2008) Perioperative events during deep brain stimulation: the experience at Cleveland Clinic. J Neurosurg Anesthesiol 20:36–40

37. Kim MS, Jung YT, Sim JH, Kim SJ, Kim JW, Burchiel KJ (2006) Microelectrode recording: lead point in STN-DBS surgery. Acta Neurochir Suppl 99:37–42
38. Kirschman DL, Milligan B, Wilkinson S, Overman J, Wetzel L, Batnitzky S et al (2000) Pallidotomy microelectrode targeting: neurophysiology-based target refinement. Neurosurgery 46:613–622
39. Klostermann F, Funk T, Vesper J, Siedenberg R, Curio G (2000) Propofol narcosis dissociates human intrathalamic and cortical high-frequency (> 400 hz) SEP components. Neuroreport 11:2607–2610
40. Klostermann F, Vesper J, Curio G (2003) Identification of target areas for deep brain stimulation in human basal ganglia substructures based on median nerve sensory evoked potential criteria. J Neurol Neurosurg Psychiatry 74:1031–1035
41. Lanotte MM, Rizzone M, Bergamasco B, Faccani G, Melcarne A, Lopiano L (2002) Deep brain stimulation of the subthalamic nucleus: anatomical, neurophysiological, and outcome correlations with the effects of stimulation. J Neurol Neurosurg Psychiatry 72:53–58
42. Lefaucheur JP, Gurruchaga JM, Pollin B, von Raison F, Mohsen N, Shin M et al (2008) Outcome of bilateral subthalamic nucleus stimulation in the treatment of Parkinson's disease: correlation with intra-operative multi-unit recordings but not with the type of anaesthesia. Eur Neurol 60:186–199
43. Lenz FA, Jaeger CJ, Seike MS, Lin YC, Reich SG, DeLong MR et al (1999) Thalamic single neuron activity in patients with dystonia: dystonia-related activity and somatic sensory reorganization. J Neurophysiol 82:2372–2392
44. Lozano AM, Hutchison WD, Tasker RR, Lang AE, Junn F, Dostrovsky JO (1998) Microelectrode recordings define the ventral posteromedial pallidotomy target. Stereotact Funct Neurosurg 71:153–163
45. Lozano AM, Kumar R, Gross RE, Giladi N, Hutchison WD, Dostrovsky JO et al (1997) Globus pallidus internus pallidotomy for generalized dystonia. Mov Disord 12:865–870
46. Lozano AM, Lang AE, Levy R, Hutchison W, Dostrovsky J (2000) Neuronal recordings in Parkinson's disease patients with dyskinesias induced by apomorphine. Ann Neurol 47:S141–S146
47. Marsden CD, Obeso JA (1994) The functions of the basal ganglia and the paradox of stereotaxic surgery in Parkinson's disease [see comments]. Brain 117:877–897
48. Morishita T, Foote KD, Wu SS, Jacobson CE, Rodriguez RL, Haq IU et al (2010) Brain penetration effects of microelectrodes and deep brain stimulation leads in ventral intermediate nucleus stimulation for essential tremor. J Neurosurg 112:491–496
49. Nandi D, Chir M, Liu X, Bain P, Parkin S, Joint C et al (2002) Electrophysiological confirmation of the zona incerta as a target for surgical treatment of disabling involuntary arm movements in multiple sclerosis: use of local field potentials. J Clin Neurosci 9:64–68
50. Oh MY, Hodaie M, Kim SH, Alkhani A, Lang AE, Lozano AM (2001) Deep brain stimulator electrodes used for lesioning: proof of principle. Neurosurgery 49:363–367
51. Ondo W, Dat VK, Almaguer M, Jankovic J, Simpson RK (2001) Thalamic deep brain stimulation: effects on the nontarget limbs. Mov Disord 16:1137–1142
52. Pierantozzi M, Mazzone P, Bassi A, Rossini PM, Peppe A, Altibrandi MG et al (1999) The effect of deep brain stimulation on the frontal N30 component of somatosensory evoked potentials in advanced Parkinson's disease patients [see comments]. Clin Neurophysiol 110:1700–1707
53. Pierantozzi M, Palmieri MG, Mazzone P, Marciani MG, Rossini PM, Stefani A et al (2002) Deep brain stimulation of both subthalamic nucleus and internal globus pallidus restores intracortical inhibition in Parkinson's disease paralleling apomorphine effects: a paired magnetic stimulation study. Clin Neurophysiol 113:108–113
54. Pinter MM, Alesch F, Murg M, Helscher RJ, Binder H (1999) Apomorphine test: a predictor for motor responsiveness to deep brain stimulation of the subthalamic nucleus. J Neurol 246:907–913
55. Pinter MM, Murg M, Alesch F, Freundl B, Helscher RJ, Binder H (1999) Does deep brain stimulation of the nucleus ventralis intermedius affect postural control and locomotion in Parkinson's disease? Mov Disord 14:958–963
56. Pinsker MO, Volkmann J, Falk D, Herzog J, Steigerwald F, Deuschl G et al (2009) Deep brain stimulation of the internal globus pallidus in dystonia: target localisation under general anaesthesia. Acta Neurochir (Wien) 151:751–758
57. Pollak P, Benabid AL, Limousin P, Benazzouz A (1997) Chronic intracerebral stimulation in Parkinson's disease. Adv Neurol 74:213–220
58. Rodriguez MC, Obeso JA, Olanow CW (1998) Subthalamic nucleus-mediated excitotoxicity in Parkinson's disease: a target for neuroprotection. Ann Neurol 44:S175–S188
59. Sansur CA, Frysinger RC, Pouratian N, Fu KM, Bittl M, Oskouian RJ et al (2007) Incidence of symptomatic hemorrhage after stereotactic electrode placement. J Neurosurg 107:998–1003
60. Schuurman PR, Bosch DA, Bossuyt PM, Bonsel GJ, van Someren EJ, de Bie RM et al (2000) A comparison of continuous thalamic stimulation and thalamotomy for suppression of severe tremor. N Engl J Med 342:461–468
61. Senatus PB, Teeple D, McClelland S III, Pullman SL, Yu Q, Ford B et al (2006) A technique for minimally altering anatomically based subthalamic electrode targeting by microelectrode recording. Neurosurg Focus 20:E8
62. Starr PA, Subramanian T, Bakay RA, Wichmann T (2000) Electrophysiological localization of the substantia nigra in the parkinsonian nonhuman primate. J Neurosurg 93:704–710
63. Starr PA, Turner RS, Rau G, Lindsey N, Heath S, Volz M et al (2004) Microelectrode-guided implantation of deep brain stimulators into the globus pallidus internus for dystonia: techniques, electrode locations, and outcomes. Neurosurg Focus 17:E4
64. Starr PA, Turner RS, Rau G, Lindsey N, Heath S, Volz M et al (2006) Microelectrode-guided implantation of deep brain stimulators into the globus pallidus internus for dystonia: techniques, electrode locations, and outcomes. J Neurosurg 104:488–501
65. Sterio D, Zonenshayn M, Mogilner AY, Rezai AR, Kiprovski K, Kelly PJ et al (2002) Neurophysiological refinement of subthalamic nucleus targeting. Neurosurgery 50:58–67
66. Struppler A, Jacobi HM, Krott HM (1969) Significance of thalamic neuronal activity in stereotaxic operations. Electroencephalogr Clin Neurophysiol 26:443–444
67. Vayssiere N, Hemm S, Zanca M, Picot MC, Bonafe A, Cif L et al (2000) Magnetic resonance imaging stereotactic target localization for deep brain stimulation in dystonic children. J Neurosurg 93:784–790
68. Venkatraghavan L, Luciano M, Manninen P (2010) Review article: anesthetic management of patients undergoing deep brain stimulator insertion. Anesth Analg 110:1138–1145
69. Vesper J, Haak S, Ostertag C, Nikkhah G (2007) Subthalamic nucleus deep brain stimulation in elderly patients – analysis of outcome and complications. BMC Neurol 7:7
70. Vesper J, Steinhoff B, Rona S, Wille C, Bilic S, Nikkhah G et al (2007) Chronic high-frequency deep brain stimulation of the STN/SNr for progressive myoclonic epilepsy. Epilepsia 48:1984–1989
71. Wichmann T, Bergman H, DeLong MR (1994) The primate subthalamic nucleus. III. Changes in motor behavior and neuronal activity in the internal pallidum induced by subthalamic inactivation in the MPTP model of parkinsonism. J Neurophysiol 72:521–530
72. Wichmann T, DeLong MR, Vitek J (2000) Pathophysiological considerations in basal ganglia surgery: role of the basal ganglia in hypokinetic and hyperkinetic movement disorders. In: Lozano AM (ed) Movement disorder surgery. Karger, Basel, pp 31–57
73. Zonenshayn M, Rezai AR, Mogilner AY, Beric A, Sterio D, Kelly PJ (2000) Comparison of anatomic and neurophysiological methods for subthalamic nucleus targeting. Neurosurgery 47:282–292

A Comparison Between Stereotactic Targeting Methods of the Subthalamic Nucleus in Cases with Parkinson's Disease

Ali Savas, Melih Bozkurt, and Cenk Akbostancı

Abstract *Background*: Several methods are used for targeting of the subthalamic nucleus (STN) for the surgical treatment of Parkinson's disease (PD). The goal of this study is to determine the most suitable morphological method for localizing the STN in order to perform deep brain stimulation (DBS) in the treatment of PD.

Methods: Twelve cases with PD underwent bilateral STN-DBS and followed up for 5 years. Indirect calculation of the STN using AC-PC coordinates, and direct targeting of the STN using stereotactic CT/MRI fusion, were used for targeting. A microelectrode recording method was used to localize the STN.

Results: Direct targeting of the STN using CT/MRI fusion was very precise in every case, based upon evaluation of the intraoperative microelectrode recordings, postoperative MRI scans, and clinical follow-up of the cases. The coordinate differences obtained from these two methods were statistically significant.

Conclusion: Direct targeting method of the STN using CT/MRI fusion provided higher precision than the indirect calculation method. This method may be used as a standard targeting technique, and may obviate the need for using complicated technologies such as microelectrode recording, which may sometimes be risky and counterproductive.

Keywords Deep brain stimulation • Subthalamic nucleus • Image fusion • Targeting • Parkinson's disease

A. Savas, MD, PhD (✉) and M. Bozkurt, MD
School of Medicine, Department of Neurosurgery, Ankara University, PK 243 Kavaklidere, Ankara 06100, Turkey
e-mail: alisavas63@yahoo.com

C. Akbostancı, MD
School of Medicine, Department of Neurology, Ankara University, PK 243 Kavaklidere, Ankara 06100, Turkey

Introduction

Deep brain stimulation (DBS) of the subthalamic nucleus (STN) is an effective surgical treatment for patients with advanced Parkinson's disease (PD). The technique of bilateral DBS of the STN has been accepted as one of the most commonly used surgical procedures since 1994, largely replacing the chronic stimulation of the ventral intermediate nucleus of the thalamus that was first reported in 1991 [4, 5, 18].

The success of STN-DBS for achieving clinical improvement is directly proportional to the accuracy of targeting the STN and lead placement [6, 22]. Different types of methods have been used to localize the STN stereotactically. The indirect coordinate calculation method using the anterior (AC) and posterior commissures (PC) has been a conventional technique for localizing the functional deep brain structures, such as the STN, thalamus, and pallidum [9, 22]. Some other methods, such as stereotactic ventriculography and direct visualization of the STN by magnetic resonance imaging (MRI), are useful for accurate localization [5, 22, 25]. Electrophysiological recording of the STN during the procedures can be applied, and provides real-time functional confirmation of the target [3, 30].

The goal of this study was to determine the most suitable morphological method to localize the STN in order to perform DBS in the treatment of cases with advanced PD.

Material and Methods

During the period 2001–2006, 12 cases (with 24 targets) with PD who underwent bilateral subthalamic DBS operations for PD were selected randomly for this study. There were seven male and five female patients. The mean age was 59.08 (44–64) years. The mean diagnosis duration was 11.1 (4–26) years, and all patients were under medical therapy on admission. Two of the patients had undergone unilateral

G. Nikkhah and M. Pinsker (eds.), *Stereotactic and Functional Neurosurgery*, Acta Neurochirurgica Supplement, Vol. 117, DOI 10.1007/978-3-7091-1482-7_6, © Springer-Verlag Wien 2013

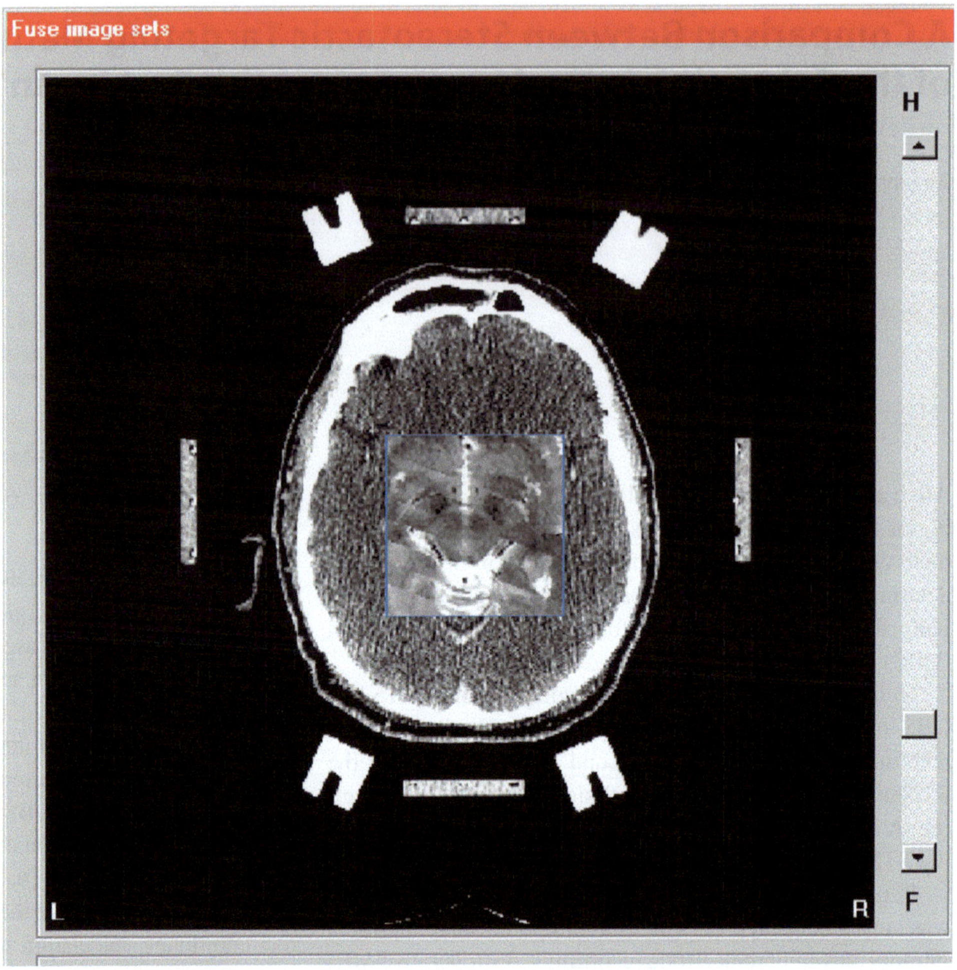

Fig. 1 Axial T2-weighted MRI data, in which the STN is visible, and CT-MRI image-fusion image

pallidotomy previously. All cases were followed for 60 months.

All surgical procedures were performed by only one neurosurgeon (AS), and all of the cases were evaluated neurologically by only one neurologist (CA). Thus, standardization of the procedures and a movement disorder protocol were established at the beginning of the study for the surgical technique, therapeutic management and neurological evaluation. Preoperatively, Unified Parkinson's Disease Rating Scale (UPDRS) scores, bradykinesia and rigidity UPDRS scores, tremor and posture UPDRS scores, Abnormal Involuntary Movement Scale (AIMS) scores, and Core Assessment Program for Intracerebral Transplantations (CAPIT) were calculated.

All of the cases were examined with brain MRI scans preoperatively without any stereotactic frame application. Axial, T2, flip angle 90°, slice thickness 1 mm, matrix 256 × 256, 1.5T MRI studies for the STN were applied to all patients. Data were analyzed with a stereotactic software program (Target@, BrainLab, Munich, Germany).

A stereotactic head ring (Riechert-Mundinger, Inomed, Emmendingen, Germany) was placed on the patients under local anesthesia. A computerized tomography (CT) was obtained under stereotactic conditions. CT-MRI image fusion and image processing were performed with the same stereotactic software.

Two different preoperative coordinate calculation methods were used for targeting the STN in all patients:

1. *The conventional indirect calculation method*: by calculating relative to the AC, PC and mid-commissural point (MCP), the STN coordinates were determined according to a brain atlas. In this method, the indirect target coordinates were calculated to target the region 3 mm posterior to the MCP, 4 mm inferior to the MCP, and 12–13 mm lateral to the AC-PC line. Left and right coordinates were evaluated separately (totally 24 coordinates).
2. *The direct calculation of the visible STN on MRI scans*: for the direct targeting of the STN, we transferred the stereotactic CT scans and the axial and coronary T2-weighted MRI data, in which the STN is visible, to our stereotactic software. We then performed CT-MRI image fusion using the stereotactic software (Fig. 1). Using this program, multiplanar reconstructions were also obtained for choosing the optimal trajectory. We then targeted the visualized

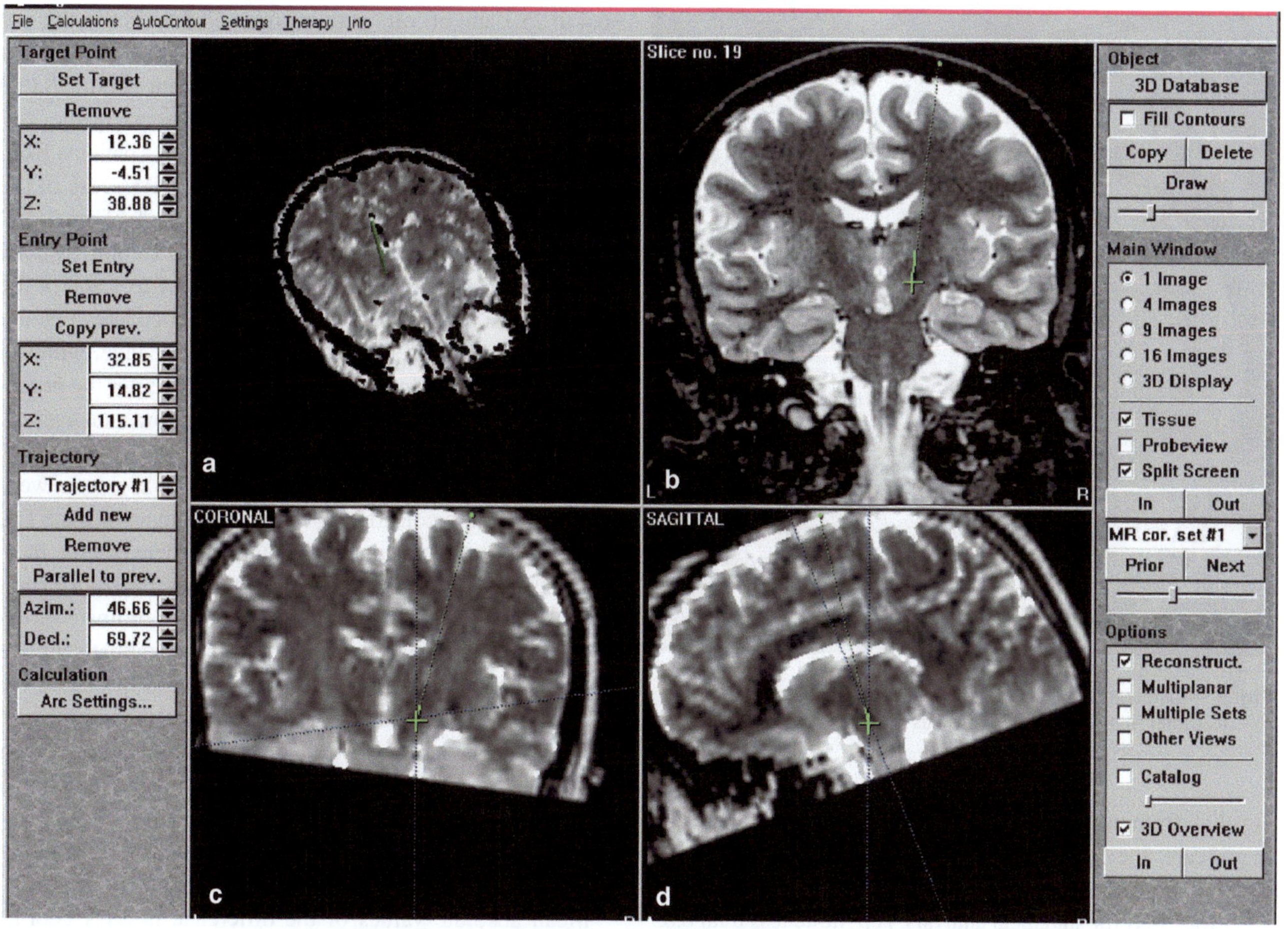

Fig. 2 Images from the multiplanar stereotactic CT-MRI image-processing program for targeting the STN and choosing the optimal trajectory. In these images, the right STN was targeted and a fronto-subthalamic trajectory was chosen just lateral to the lateral ventricle. (**a** reconstructed axial scan-trajectory image; **b** coronal-section superimposed trajectory image; **c** reconstructed coronary image parallel to the trajectory; **d** reconstructed sagittal image parallel to the trajectory)

STN, i.e., during the operative procedures, we primarily used this direct calculation method (Fig. 2).

The STN targets were also examined intra-operatively with microelectrode recording (MER) (Leadpoint$^{\text{TM}5.04}$, Medtronic, Minneapolis, MN, USA). The microstimulation technique was also used to confirm the target. A five-channel recording was started 5 mm above the calculated target and continued until 3 mm below the target, and loss of STN activity was observed.

After electrophysiological confirmation of the target, a four-contact electrode (model DBS-MRIS, Medtronic, Minneapolis, MN, USA) was implanted. All cases were examined by MRI scans after the lead implantation in order to verify the correct placement of the electrodes in the STN (Fig. 3) before the placement of the implantable pulse generator (IPG) (Kinetra, Medtronic, Minneapolis, MN, USA). One day later, the IPG was implanted subcutaneously in the subclavian area and connected to the electrodes. The monopolar electrode contacts (case positive) used for stimulation, with frequency 100–150 Hz, amplitude 2–4.5 V, and pulse width 60–120 µs, were tuned by telemetry according to the neurological responses of the patients.

All cases were followed by the Neurology Department for 5 years. Postoperative UPDRS scores, bradykinesia and rigidity UPDRS scores, tremor and posture UPDRS scores, AIMS, and CAPIT were also calculated.

STN coordinates, obtained from conventional indirect targeting and direct targeting of the STN with image-fusion technique, were compared using two methods. The coordinates calculated from the indirect method were subtracted from the direct targeting value, and the absolute values of the differences were calculated. Mean, median and standard deviation of the 24 values were calculated. 1-mm deviation for each coordinate was considered significant. Differences between the two methods for STN coordinates were evaluated by Friedman two-way analysis of variance by ranks. When the

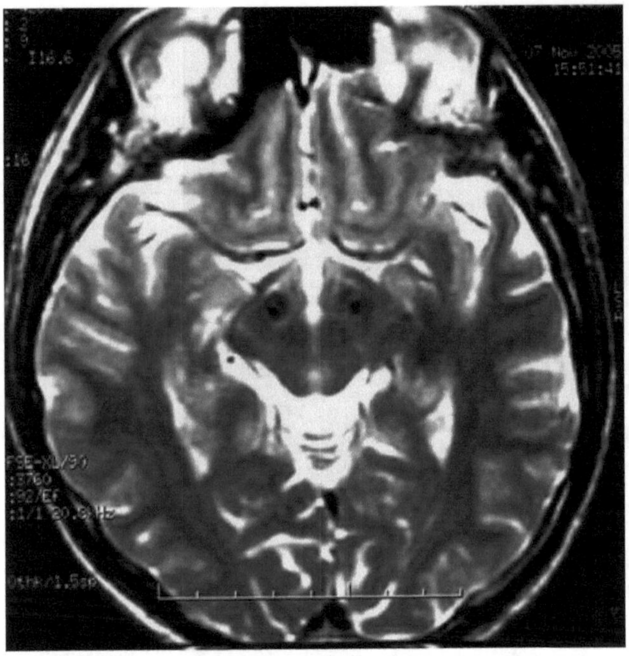

Fig. 3 Postoperative axial T2-weighted image of the patient, showing the electrodes in the subthalamic nucleus

p-value from the Friedman test statistics was statistically significant, the Bonferroni-corrected Wilcoxon signed ranks test was used to set apart the difference. SPSS for Windows 11.5 was used for statistical analysis. A *p*-value less than 0.05 was considered as significant. We also determined the deviation of STN coordinates obtained with each method using the image-fusion technique coordinates as a reference method.

$$= \sqrt{(X - Xif)^2 + (Y - Yif)^2 + (Z - Zif)^2}$$

According to the formula, if the value of the '*x*' is positive, deviation of the calculated coordinate was considered as lateral; if the value of the '*y*' is positive, deviation of the calculated coordinate was considered as anterior; and if the value of the '*z*' is positive, deviation of the calculated coordinate was considered as inferior. Using Cartesian geometry, the actual distance of the coordinates was calculated with the values from the second technique.

Results

There were no localization problems or hardware complications in the early postoperative period. No mortality was observed. No hemorrhage, infection, or any other neurological complications occurred. None of the cases had major depression, cognitive decline, or abnormalities on a MRI scan. The UPDRS score of the 'on' patients decreased from 36.4 to 25.1 and of 'off' patients from 58.5 to 38.9 at the end of the 5-year follow-up. The AIMS score of the 'on' patients decreased from 13.3 to 4.6 and of 'off' patients from 2.8 to 0 after the procedure. Bradykinesia UPDRS score of the 'on' patients decreased from 7 to 5 and of the 'off' patients from 9.4 to 7.6 after the procedure. Rigidity UPDRS score of the 'on' patients decreased from 3.3 to 1.7 and of the 'off' patients from 4.6 to 2.6 after the procedure. Tremor UPDRS score of the 'on' patients decreased from 1.1 to 1 and of the 'off' patients from 2.5 to 0.4 after the procedure. Posture UPDRS score in the 'on' patients did not change, while in the 'off' patients, it increased from 2.6 to 3.1 after the procedure. Dopaminergic drug dosage was 54 % lower on average at the end of the 5-year follow-up.

The coordinates of the STN along the *x*, *y*, *z* axes were compared. While considering the '*x*' coordinate of the STN, the deviation was calculated as significant between the indirect method and 'direct targeting' method ($p = 0.014$ for right and $p = 0.010$ for left). Considering the '*y*' coordinate of the STN, the deviation was calculated as significant between the indirect method and 'direct targeting' method ($p = 0.002$ for right and $p = 0.003$ for left). Considering the '*z*' coordinate of the STN, the deviation was calculated as significant between the indirect method and 'direct targeting' method ($p = 0.003$ for right and $p = 0.010$ for left). Data sets of the STN coordinates in the *x*-*y*-*z* axes both for indirect and direct targeting methods for individual case are summarized in Table 1.

Mean absolute values of the difference in STN coordinates between the direct versus indirect targeting were 1.6208 mm (*x* axis medial deviation), 3.8667 (*y* axis anterior deviation) and 1.908 mm (*z* axis superior deviation). Using the Cartesian geometry technique, the deviation was calculated as 4.6327 mm antero-medio-superiorly, while considering the 'direct targeting' and indirect methods.

Discussion

The STN has a critical role in the regulation of movement by transmitting the signals from the cortical areas to the output nuclei of the basal ganglia (pars reticularis of the substantia nigra (SNr) and globus pallidus interna (GPi)). The regulation is made by exerting excitatory influence with glutamate to these structures [20]. Wichmann, Guridi, and Aziz achieved amelioration of motor signs of PD by reducing STN activity using MPTP (1-methyl-4-phenyl-1,2,3,6-tetrahydropiridine) [2, 10, 29].

During the last 2 decades, DBS of the STN has become one of the main therapeutic options for medically refractory PD, and has been established as a safe and effective method by various studies [5, 8, 18]. In DBS, there is still a controversy in choosing the targeting technique to assign and

Table 1 Data set of the STN coordinates in the *x-y-z* axes both for indirect and direct targeting methods

	Indirect method		Direct method		Indirect method		Direct method		Indirect method		Direct method	
	x axis		*x* axis		*y* axis		*y* axis		*z* axis		*z* axis	
Patient number	Right	Left	Right	Left	Right	Left	Right	Left	Right	Left	Right	Left
1	8.4	−15.9	9.1	−17.2	−5.5	−5.5	−3.9	−1	33.2	33.2	28.2	38.1
2	7.3	−14.7	7.7	−18.5	−8.4	−8.4	0	4.6	32	32	28.9	32
3	3.4	−18.6	4.3	−20.2	−2.7	−2.7	−2.5	0.7	48.9	48.9	45.6	45.5
4	13.1	−10.9	10.4	−9.9	−6.1	−6.1	−3.5	−3.3	32.8	32.8	31.2	31.5
5	13.2	−10.8	11	−14	5.2	5.2	9	9.6	44.6	44.6	41.6	45.6
6	10.5	−13.5	9.7	−14.2	−1.2	−1.2	5.1	6	44.7	44.7	42.8	44.6
7	16.3	−9.7	13.7	−10.3	−3.9	−3.9	−2.2	−0.4	37.8	37.8	38	37.5
8	14.5	−11.5	11.6	−12.2	1	1	3.3	3.5	44.6	44.6	43.1	44.8
9	1	−21	−0.4	−20.7	−2.8	−2.8	−1.9	1.1	37.5	37.5	36.5	35.5
10	14	−10	12.8	−12.3	−8.4	−8.4	−4.1	−3.6	43.4	43.4	39.7	40.7
11	9.5	−14.5	12.4	−17.9	−7.2	−7.2	−2.6	−1.9	31.7	31.7	29.5	27.3
12	12.4	−11	12.4	−13.1	−5.3	−4	−4.5	−4	40	42	38.9	43.3

localize the STN. The goal of this report was to investigate the reliability of the direct targeting of the STN using CT/MRI fusion technology for accurate target localization, and to determine the difference from the conventional technique performed using the AC and PC reference points for indirect calculation. Precise localization of the STN and correct placement of the therapeutic electrodes are essential for the effectiveness of the DBS procedure [27].

Targeting the STN with CT provides rapid and accurate coordinates for stereotactic localization [24]. However, anatomic identification and discrimination of the intracranial targets are poor when compared with MRI. Especially for the STN, anatomical details are much more precisely defined by MRI [17]. On the other hand, MRI has the disadvantage of image distortion. Sumanaweera pointed to two causes of image distortion in 1994: a gradient field non-linearity and resonance offsets. They reported the causes of distortion as the fat–water ratio of the tissues and air–bone and air–tissue interactions [27]. Kondziolka compared the stereotactic coordinate determination by CT and MRI in 53 targets and for central targets, and MR-CT discrepancies were calculated as 2:09 ± 1:79. The authors explained this difference by a 1-pixel difference in target selection between the two methods [14]. Lemaire et al. reported a 1.65 mm discrepancy between MRI and CT in 83 patients undergoing thalamotomy and pallidotomy for the anterior and posterior commissures, and in 2 % of the patients, the difference was more than 4 mm [17]. Similarly, Alexander et al. calculated 4 mm three-dimensional distortion in stereotactic, frame-based MRI [1]. These results guided the authors to the conclusion that targeting based on MRI alone may not be sufficiently precise.

Direct targeting technique for the STN using CT-MRI image fusion was described previously [21]. The image-fusion procedure combines the stereotactic accuracy of CT and the precise anatomical definition of MRI. Fusion accuracy of the image-fusion procedure is equal to approximately ± 1 pixel. With the guidance of the image-fusion technique, Kooy et al. did not observe distortions greater than 1 mm except at the tissue–air interface [15]. As the red nucleus and SNr have iron contents in their structure and highly myelinated pons, the magnetic field can lead to chemical shift, and cause coordinate deviations and spatial inaccuracy [13, 19, 23]. Stereotactic frames also cause magnetic field disturbance while targeting with MRI [16]. The CT/MRI fusion technique eliminates the magnetic artifacts, coordinate deviations, and imaging problems with stereotactic frames, and stereotactic coordinates can be calculated with higher precision with a deviation of less than 1 mm or 1 pixel [28]. The precision of the STN targeting can be improved by using CT/MR fusion [7, 21].

Although many authors have reported that the DBS effect is maximized by MER mapping, electrophysiological specification of the STN margins based on the shooting pattern can be demanding because the series of steps are laborious and individual [12, 26]. Although MER has a considerable neurophysiologic value for improving the deviation of the coordinates, this technique may cause increased hematoma rates and excess operation time [11].

Our results show that the direct targeting method is rather reliable and accurate, and has a great precision. On the other hand, the coordinates obtained using the conventional indirect targeting technique showed very significant difference from those obtained from direct targeting. Thus, the indirect coordinates seem unreliable for STN targeting, and need to be corrected with other auxiliary methods such as MER. On the other hand, the direct targeting technique may obviate the need for using complicated technologies such as MER, which sometimes may be risky and counter-productive.

Conclusion

Based on our results, the STN coordinates obtained with the image-fusion technique were highly accurate, and well-correlated with clinical results and microelectrode recording. The coordinates obtained from conventional indirect targeting were significantly different from those obtained with the direct targeting technique. These results underline that direct targeting of the STN with the image-fusion technique may further improve the targeting accuracy when compared to the accuracy of the other methods.

Acknowledgement This study was abstracted from the data of a specialty thesis in neurosurgery at Ankara University School of Medicine, given by the second author (MB).

Conflict of Interest The authors declare that they have no conflict of interest.

References

1. Alexander E 3rd, Kooy HM, van Herk M, Schwartz M, Barnes PD, Tarbell N, Mulkern RV, Holupka EJ, Loeffler JS (1995) Magnetic resonance image-directed stereotactic neurosurgery: use of image fusion with computerized tomography to enhance spatial accuracy. J Neurosurg 83:271–276
2. Aziz TZ, Peggs D, Sambrook MA, Crossman AR (1991) Lesion of the subthalamic nucleus for the alleviation of 1-methyl-4-phenyl-1-,2,3,6-tetrahydropyridine (MPTP)-induced parkinsonism in the primate. Mov Disord 6:288–292
3. Bejjani BP, Dormont D, Pidoux B, Yelnik J, Damier P, Arnulf I, Bonnet AM, Marsault C, Agid Y, Philippon J, Cornu P (2000) Bilateral subthalamic stimulation for Parkinson's disease by using three-dimensional stereotactic magnetic resonance imaging and electrophysiological guidance. J Neurosurg 92:615–625

4. Benabid AL, Pollak P, Gervason C, Hoffmann D, Gao DM, Hommel M, Perret JE, de Rougemont J (1991) Long-term suppression of tremor by chronic stimulation of the ventral intermediate thalamic nucleus. Lancet 337:403–406
5. Benabid AL, Pollak P, Gross C, Hoffmann D, Benazzouz A, Gao DM, Laurent A, Gentil M, Perret J (1994) Acute and long-term effects of subthalamic nucleus stimulation in Parkinson's disease. Stereotact Funct Neurosurg 62:76–84
6. Cuny E, Guehl D, Burbaud P, Gross C, Dousset V, Rougier A (2002) Lack of agreement between direct magnetic resonance imaging and statistical determination of a subthalamic target: the role of electrophysiological guidance. J Neurosurg 97:591–597
7. Duffner F, Schiffbauer H, Breit S, Friese S, Freudenstein D (2002) Relevance of image fusion for target point determination in functional neurosurgery. Acta Neurochir 144:445–451
8. Gross RE, Lozano AM (2000) Advances in neurostimulation for movement disorders. Neurol Res 22:247–258
9. Guiot GDP, Arfel G et al (1973) Electrophysiological recordings in stereotaxic thalamotomy for parkinsonism. Prog Neurol Surg 5:189–221
10. Guridi J, Herrero MT, Luquin MR, Guillen J, Ruberg M, Laguna J, Vila M, Javoy-Agid F, Agid Y, Hirsch E, Obeso JA (1996) Subthalamotomy in parkinsonian monkeys. Behavioural and biochemical analysis. Brain 119(Pt 5):1717–1727
11. Hariz MI (2002) Complications of deep brain stimulation surgery. Mov Disord 17(Suppl 3):S162–S166
12. Kim MS, Jung YT, Sim JH, Kim SJ, Kim JW, Burchiel KJ (2006) Microelectrode recording: lead point in STN-DBS surgery. Acta Neurochir Suppl 99:37–42
13. Koeppen AH (1995) The history of iron in the brain. J Neurol Sci 134(Suppl):1–9
14. Kondziolka D, Dempsey PK, Lunsford LD, Kestle JR, Dolan EJ, Kanal E, Tasker RR (1992) A comparison between magnetic resonance imaging and computed tomography for stereotactic coordinate determination. Neurosurgery 30:402–406; discussion 406–407
15. Kooy HM, van Herk M, Barnes PD, Alexander E 3rd, Dunbar SF, Tarbell NJ, Mulkern RV, Holupka EJ, Loeffler JS (1994) Image fusion for stereotactic radiotherapy and radiosurgery treatment planning. Int J Radiat Oncol Biol Phys 28:1229–1234
16. Krauss JK, Grossman RG (2001) Principles and techniques of movement disorders surgery. In: Krauss JK, Jankovic J, Grossman RG (eds) Surgery for parkinson's disease and movement disorders. Lippincott Williams & Wilkins, Philadelphia, pp 176–187
17. Lemaire JJ, Durif F, Boire JY, Debilly B, Irthum B, Chazal J (1999) Direct stereotactic MRI location in the globus pallidus for chronic stimulation in Parkinson's disease. Acta Neurochir 141:759–765; discussion 766
18. Limousin P, Pollak P, Benazzouz A, Hoffmann D, Le Bas JF, Broussolle E, Perret JE, Benabid AL (1995) Effect of parkinsonian signs and symptoms of bilateral subthalamic nucleus stimulation. Lancet 345:91–95
19. Novak P, Novak V, Kangarlu A, Abduljalil AM, Chakeres DW, Robitaille PM (2001) High resolution MRI of the brainstem at 8T. J Comput Assist Tomogr 25:242–246
20. Parent A, Hazrati LN (1995) Functional anatomy of the basal ganglia. II. The place of subthalamic nucleus and external pallidum in basal ganglia circuitry. Brain research. Brain Res Rev 20:128–154
21. Savas AAC, Yagmurlu B, Elibol B, Erden I, Kanpolat Y (2002) A new method for subthalamic nucleus targeting using CT/MRI image-fusion technology. Acta Neurochir 144:1076–1077
22. Schaltenbrand G, Wahren W (1997) Atlas for sterotaxy of the human brain. Thime Verlag, Stuttgart
23. Smith RC, Lange RC, McCarthy SM (1991) Chemical shift artifact: dependence on shape and orientation of the lipid-water interface. Radiology 181:225–229
24. Spiegelmann R, Friedman WA (1991) Rapid determination of thalamic CT-stereotactic coordinates: a method. Acta Neurochir 110:77–81
25. Starr PA (2002) Placement of deep brain stimulators into the subthalamic nucleus or globus pallidus internus: technical approach. Stereotact Funct Neurosurg 79:118–145
26. Sterio D, Zonenshayn M, Mogilner AY, Rezai AR, Kiprovski K, Kelly PJ, Beric A (2002) Neurophysiological refinement of subthalamic nucleus targeting. Neurosurgery 50:58–67; discussion 67–59
27. Sumanaweera TS, Adler JR Jr, Napel S, Glover GH (1994) Characterization of spatial distortion in magnetic resonance imaging and its implications for stereotactic surgery. Neurosurgery 35:696–703; discussion 703–694
28. Voges J, Volkmann J, Allert N, Lehrke R, Koulousakis A, Freund HJ, Sturm V (2002) Bilateral high-frequency stimulation in the subthalamic nucleus for the treatment of parkinson disease: correlation of therapeutic effect with anatomical electrode position. J Neurosurg 96:269–279
29. Wichmann T, Bergman H, DeLong MR (1994) The primate subthalamic nucleus. III. Changes in motor behavior and neuronal activity in the internal pallidum induced by subthalamic inactivation in the MPTP model of parkinsonism. J Neurophysiol 72:521–530
30. Zonenshayn M, Rezai AR, Mogilner AY, Beric A, Sterio D, Kelly PJ (2000) Comparison of anatomic and neurophysiological methods for subthalamic nucleus targeting. Neurosurgery 47:282–292; discussion 292–284

Behind the Screen: Pseudobulbar Symptoms After Deep Brain Stimulation

Florian Amtage, Johann Lambeck, Sebastian Rutsch, Thomas Prokop, Marcus Pinsker, and Michel Rijntjes

Abstract *Background*: Thalamotomy was formerly used to treat different tremor syndromes. Nowadays, deep brain stimulation has become an established technique to treat different movement disorders. The combination of these two stereotactic interventions is rare. *Clinical Presentation*: We present a patient in which a right-sided tremor syndrome with an underlying pathology of combined essential tremor and Parkinsonian tremor was successfully treated initially with a left-sided thalamotomy and subsequently with bilateral deep brain stimulation in the subthalamic nucleus. *Results*: Deep brain stimulation in the subthalamic nucleus resulted in hemidystonia, pathological laughing and crying, dysarthria and dysphagia, all due to dislocation of the stimulation electrodes contacting the internal capsule. After discontinuation of the high-frequency stimulation these side-effects disappeared, but were then reactivated by an LCD television in stand-by mode. *Conclusion*: In this report we discuss the pathophysiology of pseudobulbar symptoms and pathological laughing and crying in context of thalamotomy and dislocated DBS electrodes. Furthermore, we report on the occurrence that magnetic fields in the household have an impact on deep brain stimulation, even if they are in stand-by mode.

F. Amtage, MD (✉), J. Lambeck, S. Rutsch, and M. Rijntjes
Department of Neurology, University Medical Center Freiburg, Breisacherstr. 64, Freiburg 79106, Germany
e-mail: florian.amtage@uniklinik-freiburg.de

T. Prokop
Division of Stereotactic and Functional Neurosurgery, University Medical Center Freiburg, Breisacherstr. 64, Freiburg 79106, Germany

M. Pinsker, MD
Department of General Neurosurgery, Neurosurgical Clinic, University Medical Center Freiburg, Breisacher Straße 64, Freiburg D-79106, Germany

Klinik für Neurochirurgie, HELIOS Klinikum Berlin-Buch, Schwanebecker Chaussee 50, Berlin DE-13125, Germany

Keywords Deep brain stimulation • Thalamotomy • Subthalamic nucleus • Pathological laughing and crying • Pseudobulbar • Parkinson's disease • Television

Introduction

Pseudobulbar symptoms such as pathologic laughing and crying (PLC), an uncontrolled expression of emotions without an appropriate trigger, are a rare complication of deep brain stimulation (DBS) in the subthalamic nucleus (STN). The pathophysiology of this phenomenon, and the anatomical structures involved, are still under debate: however, new findings suggest a disruption of cortico-ponto-cerebellar circuits [8, 9].

We report on a patient with a right-sided tremor syndrome which was treated by left-sided thalamotomy and later on by DBS of the STN due to emerging Parkinson's disease, featuring pseudobulbar symptoms and hemidystonia due to dislocation of DBS electrodes and high-frequency stimulation of the internal capsule. After switching off the stimulating system, the stimulator was reactivated by a LCD television in stand-by mode, producing these side-effects again.

Case Presentation

A 59-year-old female was admitted to our hospital in 1998 for clinical diagnostics and treatment of a progressive, right-accentuated tremor syndrome. Clinically, the right-sided tremor syndrome consisted of resting, postural, and intentional tremor, whereas on the left side solely a postural tremor was visible. Tremor analysis via both electromyography of the flexor and extensor muscles of the wrist and accelerometer recording revealed a right-sided central tremor pattern with a resting tremor frequency at 4.0 Hz and a postural

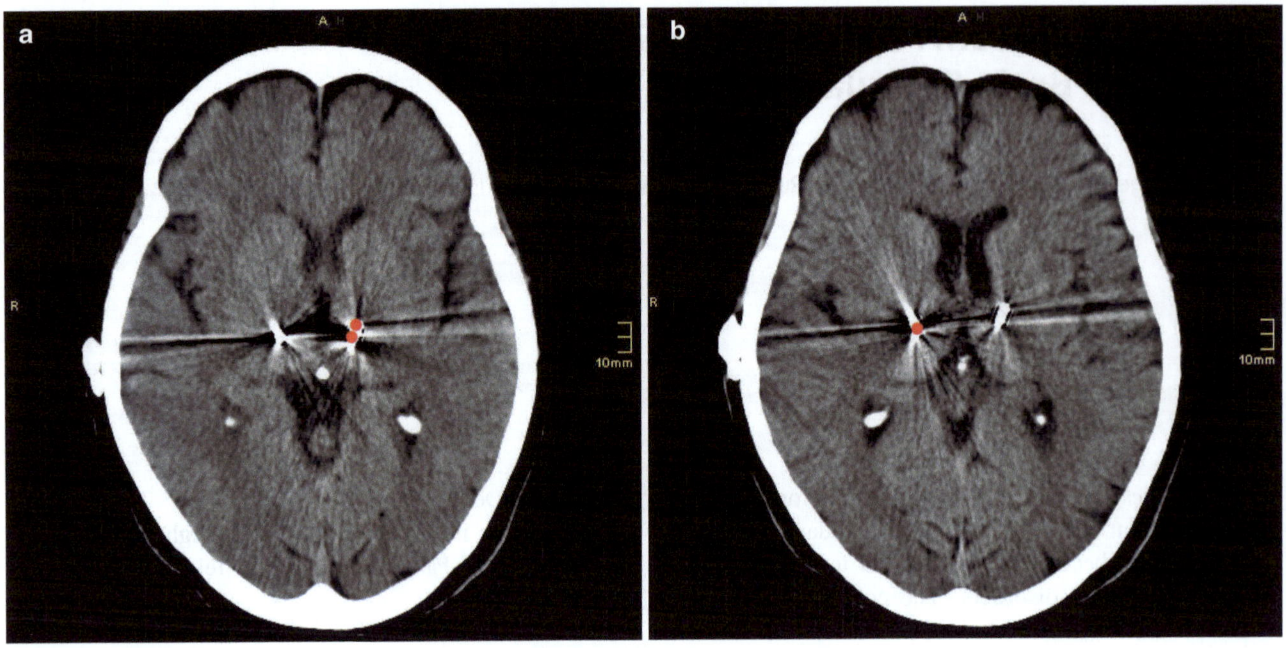

Fig. 1 Transversal slices of the computed tomography of this patient with *red circles* indicating the stimulated contacts. (**a**) Transversal slice in plane with the AC-PC-line. (**b**) Transversal slice 3 mm dorsal to the AC-PC-line

tremor frequency at 4.1 Hz. The left-sided postural tremor had a frequency at 4.1 Hz.

Based on the patient's history, the tremor syndrome started in adolescence as a bilateral postural tremor accentuated in the right upper limb, with a positive family history (mother, grandfather) and a good response to ethanol. Over time, the patient developed a right-sided intention tremor, all together consistent with the diagnosis of an essential tremor (ET). Two years before admission, an additional right-sided resting tremor occurred, suggesting a superimposed Parkinsonian tremor.

A secondary tremor syndrome was ruled out by an unremarkable magnet resonance imaging. ^{123}Iodobenzamide (IBZM-)SPECT and ^{18}FDG-PET were rated as normal. For treatment of the right-sided tremor, the patient underwent a left-sided thalamotomy. Post-thalamotomy FDG-PET revealed the expected hypometabolism of the left thalamus and, furthermore, a hypometabolism in frontal, parietal, and temporal parts of the left hemisphere, corresponding to the cortical projections of the ventro-lateral thalamus. In addition, hypometabolism of the right cerebellar hemisphere was detected. In 1999, presynaptic dopamine transporter labelling with FP-CIT revealed left-sided nigrostriatal neurodegeneration, confirming the suspected diagnosis of an idiopathic Parkinson's disease (PD).

In 2002, stereotactic bilateral implantation of DBS electrodes targeting the STN (Kinetra® 7428 Neurostimulator, DBS leads 3389; Medtronic Inc., Minneapolis, MN, USA) was performed at an external neurosurgical department for treatment of progressive PD. Postoperatively, the patient complained of slight dysarthria and dystonia in the right leg under stimulation. By increasing the amplitude several years later, the patient displayed right-sided hemidystonia and aggravation of the dysarthria, in combination with pseudobulbar signs such as dysphagia and PLC.

In 2009, the patient admitted herself to our hospital for a second opinion. Cranial computed tomography revealed a dislocation of the left-sided electrode (Fig. 1a), leading to a stimulation of the medial parts of the internal capsule with the two uppermost contacts (3.5 V, 60 μs, 150 Hz; 12.5 mm lateral, 3 mm posterior, 0 mm inferior of Mid-AC-PC-point). In addition, the right-sided electrode (Fig. 1b) was placed in a pronounced dorsolateral position (14.5 mm lateral, 3.5 mm posterior and 1 mm superior to the Mid-AC-PC-point), stimulating the internal capsule at low amplitude at the second proximal contact (0.8 V, 60 μs, 150 Hz). Testing of the remaining contacts for therapeutic effect showed no benefit to the PD symptoms. We hence turned off the neurostimulator with the patient's therapy controller (Access™, Medtronic Inc., Minneapolis, MN, USA) and increased the medication for PD. The patient's right-sided tremor was still well-controlled due to the thalamotomy performed 10 years earlier, and only a slight right-sided intention tremor and left-sided postural tremor were observed during clinical examination. Dysarthria, dysphagia, and PLC as well as the right-sided hemidystonia disappeared completely. The patient was satisfied with this outcome, and subsequently discharged from hospital. A revision of the electrodes was offered to the patient. She denied an intervention, experiencing well-being under medication after the relief of the distracting side-effects.

One month later, the patient again called for advice, since the pseudobulbar symptoms had reappeared during housework. Once again, the patient presented with right-sided hemidystonia and showed identical pseudobulbar symptoms (dysarthria, dysphagia, PLC). An assessment of the neurostimulator revealed that high-frequency stimulation was again provoking these symptoms, while the amplitude of the right stimulation contact was still set to zero. The patient insisted that the stimulation was restarted neither by herself nor by any other physician. When asked for further details about the housework, she reported that the symptoms suddenly reappeared while leaning over her television screen (LCD TV, HD-ready, Funai, Japan) — which was in stand-by mode — to dust its back cover. Therefore, the magnetic field of the television interfered with the stimulator and switched it on again, since we had neglected to inactivate the magnetic switch of the stimulator, or to set the amplitude of the left-sided stimulation parameters to zero after switching off the stimulation with the patient's controller. After deactivating the stimulator, the pseudobulbar signs promptly disappeared again.

Discussion

In addition to PLC, our patient showed more pseudobulbar symptoms such as dysphagia and dysarthria, due to dislocation of both DBS stimulation leads into the internal capsule. Moreover, a hemidystonic syndrome was provoked by the high-frequency stimulation of the cortico-spinal tract within the left internal capsule. This is in accordance with the pathophysiological concept proposed by Parvizi et al., where a disruption to the cortico-ponto-cerebellar pathway leads to PLC [8]. This would explain PLC after high-frequency stimulation of the caudal internal capsule, which directly affects the cortico-bulbar pathway [6]. Using [18F]fluorodeoxyglucose (18FDG-)PET in a patient with PLC, Wojtecki et al. [10] observed upon stimulation of the uppermost contact an activation of the ipsilateral thalamus and pons, as well as the contralateral cerebellum: this suggested an impact on the internal capsule [10].

As in two other cases with PLC after DBS [7, 10] we suggest a concomitant vulnerability of this circuit due to left-sided thalamotomy, as documented by the FDG-PET findings after thalamotomy, since only rarely patients with side-effects such as hemidystonia or spasticity also present with PLC due to high-frequency stimulation of the internal capsule. The thalamotomy in 1998 was very successful in terms of promoting a long-lasting effect on tremor reduction. Post-interventional FDG-PET revealed hypometabolism of the cortical projection areas of the ventro-lateral thalamus as well as the contralateral cerebellum. While the findings related to the cortical hypometabolism confirm previous reports after thalamotomy [1, 5], this is the first report showing a reduction in contralateral cerebellar function. The pattern of cortical glucose hypometabolism after thalamotomy is indicative of disruption of the cerebello-thalamo-cortical pathway at thalamic level, leaving the contralateral cerebellar hypometabolism unexplained. As there is no direct feedback from the thalamus to the cerebellum, an antidromic effect after thalamic stimulation has been proposed [2]. Since tremor activity is conducted via the sensorimotor cortex [3, 4], it is more likely that the cortical hypometabolism induced by thalamotomy results in a contralateral cerebellar dysfunction via reduced cortico-ponto-cerebellar output. Nevertheless, the left-sided thalamotomy was not able to provoke PLC by itself; only additional high-frequency stimulation of the internal capsule resulted in PLC and other pseudobulbar symptoms. Furthermore, the right-sided stimulation of the internal capsule did not produce a clinically-apparent dystonia, but rather spasticity of the left leg, since stimulation of only a small amplitude was applied. In addition, switching off the right-sided stimulation yielded no benefit with respect to the PLC, suggesting that bilateral pathology is therefore not mandatory to provoke PLC. This is in line with one report, showing PLC after left-sided pallidotomy and left sided STN-DBS, confirming that unilateral pathology causes PLC [7].

The magnetic field of a 3-year-old LCD television in stand-by mode was sufficient to reactivate the DBS stimulator via its magnetic switch. It seems remarkable that even small magnetic fields in the household can influence the stimulation process. Thus, we recommend, as a general rule, inactivating the magnetic switch. A permanent deactivation of the stimulation system must be achieved by setting the amplitude of the stimulator to zero so that even when a magnetic field does reactivate the stimulator, no effective stimulation is applied.

In this case, a revision of the DBS leads was indicated, and offered to the patient, but she denied a further intervention. This put a question mark on the primary indication to DBS for treatment of Parkinson's disease, but might be explained by the long time period between implantation and deactivation if the dopaminergic therapy was reduced. Therefore, the therapeutic window for a good motor response to dopaminergic therapy expands, leading to a more effective medical treatment after deactivation of the stimulator, giving no necessity for a surgical revision.

Conclusion

The occurrence of pseudobulbar symptoms in patients with DBS of the STN should prompt verification of both the anatomical location of the stimulation leads and the presence of accompanying lesions that might disturb the cortico-ponto-cerebellar pathway. Secondly, the magnetic switch of the stimulator has to be switched off as a routine procedure, since even small magnetic fields in the household can interfere with the stimulator.

Acknowledgment Many thanks for helpful comments on the manuscript to Dr. Sandra Dieni.

Conflict of Interest We declare that we have no conflict of interest.

References

1. Boecker H, Wills AJ, Ceballos-Baumann A, Samuel M, Thomas DG, Marsden CD, Brooks DJ (1997) Stereotactic thalamotomy in tremor-dominant Parkinson's disease: an H2(15)O PET motor activation study. Ann Neurol 41:108–111
2. Deiber MP, Pollak P, Passingham R, Landais P, Gervason C, Cinotti L, Friston K, Frackowiak R, Mauguiere F, Benabid AL (1993) Thalamic stimulation and suppression of parkinsonian tremor. Evidence of a cerebellar deactivation using positron emission tomography. Brain 116:267–279
3. Hellwig B, Häussler S, Lauk M, Guschlbauer B, Köster B, Kristeva-Feige R, Timmer J, Lücking CH (2000) Tremor-correlated cortical activity detected by electroencephalography. Clin Neurophysiol 111:806–809
4. Hellwig B, Häussler S, Schelter B, Lauk M, Guschlbauer B, Timmer J, Lücking CH (2001) Tremor-correlated cortical activity in essential tremor. Lancet 357:519–523
5. Henselmans JM, de Jong BM, Pruim J, Staal MJ, Rutgers AW, Haaxma R (2000) Acute effects of thalamotomy and pallidotomy on regional cerebral metabolism, evaluated by PET. Clin Neurol Neurosurg 102:84–90
6. Low HL, Sayer FT, Honey CR (2008) Pathological crying caused by high-frequency stimulation in the region of the caudal internal capsule. Arch Neurol 65:264–266
7. Okun MS, Raju DV, Walter BL, Juncos JL, DeLong MR, Heilman K, McDonald WM, Vitek JL (2004) Pseudobulbar crying induced by stimulation in the region of the subthalamic nucleus. J Neurol Neurosurg Psychiatry 75:921–923
8. Parvizi J, Anderson SW, Martin CO, Damasio H, Damasio AR (2001) Pathological laughter and crying: a link to the cerebellum. Brain 124:1708–1719
9. Parvizi J, Coburn KL, Shillcutt SD, Coffey CE, Lauterbach EC, Mendez MF (2009) Neuroanatomy of pathological laughing and crying: a report of the American Neuropsychiatric Association Committee on Research. J Neuropsychiatry Clin Neurosci 21: 75–87
10. Wojtecki L, Nickel J, Timmermann L, Maarouf M, Sudmeyer M, Schneider F, Seitz RJ, Voges J, Sturm V, Schnitzler A (2007) Pathological crying induced by deep brain stimulation. Mov Disord 22:1314–1316

Psychiatric Side-Effects of Bilateral Deep Brain Stimulation for Movement Disorders

Marcus Pinsker, Florian Amtage, Mathias Berger, Guido Nikkhah, and Ludger Tebartz van Elst

Abstract *Introduction*: The effects of deep brain stimulation (DBS) on cognitive functions, and its psychiatric side-effects, are still controversial. The present study investigated psychiatric comorbidity and postoperative effects of DBS of different targets on mood and psychological functions in 81 patients with a mean follow-up of 37 months.

Methods: A total of 109 patients underwent implantation of DBS electrodes between 2001 and 2006; it was possible to evaluate 81 patients by a psychiatric test battery using the "Neuropsychiatric Inventory". To evaluate the possible influence of the target, we analyzed the data without 16 patients with DBS surgery for other diseases (e.g., epilepsia, cluster headache) or unilateral implantation only. The resulting population (n=65, mean age 61 years, range 23–78 years, male:female 42:23) consisted of 43 Parkinson's disease patients stimulated in the subthalamic nucleus, ten dystonia patients stimulated in the globus pallidus internus, and 12 tremor patients in the ventral intermediate nucleus.

Results: There was a high rate of preoperative psychiatric comorbidity, which is reflected by a high rate of patients with preoperative medication of neuroleptic drugs (18.4 %, especially clozapin 14.7 %) and antidepressive drugs (16.5 %). Depression was the most common psychiatric side-effect after DBS, occurring in 47.7 % of all patients (31/65 patients), without significant preference to a specific target (STN: 42 %, Gpi: 60 %, VIM: 58 %). Delusion (n=5 out of 43 PD patients, 11.6 %), euphoria (n=1, 2.3 %) and disinhibition (n=3, 7.0 %) were seen in the PD patients only.

Conclusion: A wide range of behavioural changes may be seen following DBS. Depression was the most common side-effect after DBS, and occurred independently of the target. PD patients, in contrast to dystonia and tremor patients, developed complications in all tested subgroups, with varying frequencies. Preoperative evaluation for psychiatric and cognitive dysfunction is crucial to identify patients who are at specific risk for psychiatric complications.

Keywords Deep brain stimulation • Movement disorders • Psychiatric side-effects

M. Pinsker, MD (✉)
Division of Stereotactic and Functional Neurosurgery,
Department of General Neurosurgery, Neurosurgical Clinic,
University Medical Center Freiburg,
Breisacher Straße 64, Freiburg D-79106, Germany

Klinik für Neurochirurgie, HELIOS Klinikum Berlin-Buch,
Schwanebecker Chaussee 50, Berlin DE-13125, Germany
e-mail: marcus.pinsker@helios-kliniken.de

F. Amtage, MD
Department of Neurology,
University Medical Center Freiburg,
Breisacher Straße 64, Freiburg D-79106, Germany

M. Berger, MD, PhD and L. Tebartz van Elst, MD, PhD
Department of Psychiatry, University Medical Center Freiburg,
Freiburg, Germany

G. Nikkhah, MD, PhD
Division of Stereotactic and Functional Neurosurgery,
Department of General Neurosurgery, Neurosurgical Clinic,
University Medical Center Freiburg,
Breisacher Straße 64, Freiburg D-79106, Germany

Neurosurgical Clinic,
University Hospital Erlangen,
Schwabachanlage 6, Erlangen D-91054, Germany
e-email: guido.nikkhah@uk-erlangen.de

Introduction

The effectiveness of deep brain stimulation (DBS) regarding the improvement of motor function and on the quality of life (QoL) has been shown in prospective, randomized studies for Parkinson's disease (PD) [1, 2] and dystonia [3, 4]. On the other hand, the effects of DBS on cognitive functions and its psychiatric side-effects are still controversial [5], and there are several neuropsychological studies reporting a decline in executive functioning, especially in verbal fluency tasks after DBS [6–8].

G. Nikkhah and M. Pinsker (eds.), *Stereotactic and Functional Neurosurgery*, Acta Neurochirurgica Supplement, Vol. 117,
DOI 10.1007/978-3-7091-1482-7_8, © Springer-Verlag Wien 2013

The present study evaluates preoperative prevalence of psychiatric symptoms among a series of 81 out of 109 patients consecutively operated with DBS for different indications, and the effects of bilateral DBS of the subthalamic nucleus (STN), the globus pallidus internus (GPI), and the ventral intermedius nucleus (VIM) of the thalamus on mood and psychological functions in 65 patients with PD (n=43; STN bilateral), dystonia (n=10, GPI bilateral) and tremor (n=12, VIM bilateral) with a mean follow-up of 37 months, taking into account the frequency of psychiatric disturbances before and after surgery, their relation to the specific target being stimulated, and the influence of the duration of the stimulation.

Methods and Materials

Clinical Characteristics of All Patients

Files of all patients (n=109) being operated between 2001 and 2006 were analyzed retrospectively focused on notes concerning psychiatric and non-psychiatric non-motor symptoms, visits of psychiatric physicians, medication, previous brain surgery, encephalitis, or symptoms of dementia. Eighty-one out of 109 patients agreed to be further evaluated by the psychiatric test battery postoperatively. A total of 28 patients could not be evaluated due to different reasons (ten patients lived abroad and came just for the operation to our department; 13 patients did not answer, four patients were deceased, one patient could not perform the test due to deafness). Targets were the subthalamic nucleus in 43 patients, the internal globus pallidus in ten patients, and the ventral intermedius nucleus of the thalamus in another 12 patients. In 16 out of the 81 patients DBS was performed unilaterally or due to other indications, e.g., cluster headache or epilepsy. Therefore, a group of 65 patients could be evaluated with regard to the influence of bilateral DBS in different targets on psychiatric outcome. Mean age of the whole patient group (n=81) eligible for the evaluation was 59.9 years, range from 23 to 78 years; male to female ratio was 53:28. The majority (n=67, 82.7 %) was retired; only nine patients (11.1 %) were still employed, another two patients (2.5 %) were certified unfit for work.

Neuropsychiatric Assessment

For evaluation of the postoperative psychiatric symptoms, we used the Neuropsychiatric Inventory (NPI) — an instrument for assessment of neuropsychiatric symptoms in patients with neurologic disorders [9]. This instrument is well-validated and -established for the assessment of neuropsychiatric symptoms in the context of movement disorders [10, 11]. The NPI is a caregiver-based instrument which assesses the following behavioural domains in patients with neurological diseases: delusion, hallucinations, agitation/aggression, depression, anxiety, euphoria, apathy, disinhibition, irritability, aberrant motor activity, behaviour at night, and behaviour while eating. The test evaluates the presence of a specific symptom, how often it occurs (up to 4 points; e.g., once per week or daily), and the symptom severity (up to 3 points). The maximum score for each item is $4\times3=12$ points, the minimum is $1\times1=1$ point; higher scores indicate more severe and more frequent symptoms. In addition to the administration of NPI, patients were asked to judge the effect of the procedure on a scale of −5 (very bad compared to the preoperative status) to +5 (excellent compared to the preoperative status). Finally, they were asked in an open question to judge if in hindsight they would opt for the operation again or if they rather wouldn't have chosen this option. The mean duration between surgery and the test procedure was 37.4 months (PD), 32.2 months (dystonia) and 42.9 months (tremor).

Surgical Procedure

The implantation of the deep brain stimulation electrodes into the STN, GPI, or VIM was performed bilaterally during a single procedure under local anaesthesia. The target coordinates were determined on the basis of stereotactic computed tomography and intraoperative image fusion with a three-dimensional MRI. Microelectrode recording and intraoperative test stimulation was used in all patients to identify the region with best clinical effect and fewest stimulation-related side-effects. The Kinetra™ pulse generator was implanted on the same day, or the day after, under general anaesthesia. Stimulation was started within 1–3 days after surgery using monopolar settings. The postoperative standard pulse setting was 60 μs at 130 Hz; the voltage and the doses of medications were adjusted in the months following surgery in order to optimize clinical benefit.

Results

Preoperative Psychiatric Morbidity

Mean age of all NPI patients was 59.9 years, with a range of 23–78 years. Among this group, there was a high rate of patients on regular medication with neuroleptic drugs (18.4 %), especially clozapin (14.7 %) and antidepressive drugs (16.5 %). Depressive symptoms were found in 18 patients (22.2 %), psychotic symptoms in four patients (4.9 %), cognitive symptoms in six patients (7.4 %) and mania in two patients (2.5 %). Thus, at baseline, i.e., prior to implantation of a deep brain stimulator, there was a high prevalence of psychiatric symptoms, with a focus on depressive symptoms. However, 49 patients (60.5 %) were without signs of psychiatric disorders according to the medical records.

It is remarkable that Parkinson patients had a 10-fold increased prevalence of displaying symptoms of a dementia in our study group, with five out of 46 patients (10.9 %) being affected, compared to a prevalence of less than 1 % in the comparable age group of the general population [12].

Postoperative Psychiatric Symptoms

The frequency of postoperative psychiatric symptoms in relation to the three different targets is shown in Table 1. Depression, regarding to the NPI testing, was observed in 49.4 % ($n=40$) of all patients following DBS. Interestingly there was no significant preference to a specific target (STN: 18/24, 42 %; GPI: 6/10, 60 %; VIM: 7/12, 58 %). Delusions ($n=5$ out of 43 PD patients, 11.6 %), euphoria ($n=1$, 2.3 %) and disinhibition ($n=3$, 7.0 %) were seen in the PD patients only.

Correlation between duration of DBS and intensity of psychiatric symptoms showed a trend for the item apathy ($r=0.507$; $p=0.064$), which means that patients had a more intense occurrence of these symptoms than patients with shorter duration of DBS.

The item irritability was found to have a correlation for the NPI total score ($r=0.400$; $p=0.026$) and for the dynamic ($r=0.561$; $p=0.001$) of the psychopathology, which means that both severity and postoperative deterioration were related to the duration of deep brain stimulation.

Patients' Satisfaction

In line with the NPI interview, the patients were asked if they would choose the operation again as a treatment option. Results are shown in Table 2. Overall, the majority of patients ($n=58$, 72 %) was satisfied with the result and would choose the surgical treatment again. The main reason for rejection of this option was disappointment with clinical outcome; in three cases, the postoperative course was complicated by an infection. In three cases, the psychiatric side-effects were mentioned as a reason for rejection from a retrospective point of view.

To summarize the most relevant findings, in about 40 % of the patients we found psychiatric symptoms before the operation, most frequently a depression, which was more frequent compared to the general population. NPI showed that the prevalence of depressive symptoms following a DBS procedure can be up to 50 %, followed by irritability with up to 40 %, and aberrant behaviour at night 20 %. There were no differences between different targets and indications (STN, GPI, VIM). A significant correlation between intensity and clinical progress of the symptom and duration of stimulation

Table 1 Frequency of postoperative psychiatric symptoms in relation to the target evaluated with the NPI

	Frequency						
NPI- item	STN	GPI	VIM	Total	Chi-square	df	*P*
Delusion					2.771	2	0.250
Existent	5	0	0	5			
Non-existent	38	10	12	60			
Hallucination					1.462	2	0.481
Existent	9	1	1	11			
Non-existent	34	9	11	54			
Agitation/ aggression					2.904	4	0.574
Existent	6	2	0	8			
Non-existent	36	8	12	56			
n.a.	1	0	0	1			
Depression					2.061	4	0.725
Existent	18	6	7	31			
Non-existent	24	4	5	33			
n.a.	1	0	0	1			
Anxiety					1.057	2	0.589
Existent	4	2	1	7			
Non-existent	39	8	11	58			
Euphoria					0.520	2	0.771
Existent	1	0	0	1			
Non-existent	42	10	12	64			
Apathy					2.680	2	0.262
Existent	8	0	3	11			
Non-existent	35	10	10	54			
Disinhibition					1.609	2	0.447
Existent	3	0	0	3			
Non-existent	40	10	12	62			
Irritability					1.139	2	0.566
Existent	18	4	3	25			
Non-existent	25	6	9	40			
Aberrant motor activity					0.520	2	0.771
Existent	1	0	0	1			
Non-existent	42	10	12	64			
Behaviour at night					0.483	2	0.785
Existent	11	2	2	50			
Non-existent	32	8	10	15			
Behaviour while eating					2.362	2	0.307
Existent	7	1	0	8			
Non-existent	36	9	12	57			

Table 2 Patient's satisfaction with surgery

DBS again?	PD	Dyst	Tremor	Other	Total
No	8	2	6	2	18 (22 %)
Yes	35	9	12	2	58 (72 %)
I don't know	2	2	0	0	4 (5 %)
n.a.	1	0	0	0	1 (1 %)
Total	46	13	18	4	81

was found for the item irritability. Most patients would choose the procedure again due to the clinical benefit.

Discussion

Deep brain stimulation is a surgical treatment for certain types of otherwise treatment-resistant movement disorders. Positive effects are improvement in motor scores in 98.2 % [13], improvements in quality of life [1], and reduction of medication combined with reduction of medication-related side-effects. However, the frequency of psychiatric side-effects of DBS in patients with movement disorders is still a controversial debate. In a meta-analysis by Appleby et al. [13] covering the time period from Jan 1996 to Dec 2005, 808 articles out of a total of 2,667 were included for further analysis with respect to psychiatric and neuropsychiatric adverse events associated with deep brain stimulation. Overall, the prevalence of depression was 2–4 %, mania 0.9–1.7 %, and emotional changes 0.1–0.2 %. Prevalence of suicidal ideation/suicide attempt was 0.3–0.7 %, completed suicide rate was 0.16–0.32 %. The reported rates for depression, cognitive impairment, mania and behavioural change were low; however, most of the reviewed articles focused on improvement of motor function and device- or procedure-related side-effects. For example, only 18 studies reported impact of DBS on the mentation, behaviour, and mood (MBM) scale (improvement in ten, worsening in six, no change in two studies).

Witt et al. [14] presented data from a randomised, multicentre study of PD patients. Ten of 60 DBS patients had severe psychiatric side-effects (one suicide, four depression, four psychosis, one apathy), compared to 8/63 patients (one death in psychotic episode, one psychosis) in the best medical treatment group. Deep brain stimulation did not reduce overall cognition or affectivity, although there was a selective decrease in frontal cognitive functions, especially in verbal fluency (which did not affect improvements in quality of life in those patients affected). Daniels et al. [15] presented risk factors for executive dysfunction after subthalamic nucleus stimulation in Parkinson's disease from the same randomized patient population as Witt et al. [14]. Change scores were calculated for the cognitive domains "global cognitive functioning", "memory", "working memory", "attention", and "executive function", and were correlated with previously defined preoperative parameters. Compared with the BMT group, the STN-DBS group showed a significant decline only in the domain "executive function" 6 months after DBS, which was significantly correlated with age, levodopa-equivalence dosage (LED) and axial subscore of the UPDRS in the off-medication state at baseline. However, these three factors explained only about 23 % of the variance in multiple regression analysis, so other factors e.g., surgical procedure, exact placement of the electrode, or the postsurgical management might be more relevant for a decline in executive functioning after STN-DBS.

Parsons et al. [7] published a meta-analysis of 28 cohort studies (including 612 patients) from 1990 to 2006. Moderate declines were only reported in semantic (Cohen's d 0.73) and phonemic verbal fluency (0.51). Changes in verbal fluency were not related to patient age, disease duration, stimulation parameters, or change in dopamine-mimetic dose after surgery. In their conclusion, STN-DBS seemed safe in selected patients from a cognitive point of view. The difficulties in identification of factors underlying changes in verbal fluency draw attention to the need for uniform and detailed further studies on that issue.

Depression is one of the most frequent psychiatric symptoms in the general population, with an incidence of about 1 %, and is even more frequent in PD patients with up to 33.6 % [16]. There are only a small number of epidemiologic studies concerning the frequency of complication of Parkinson's disease by dementia, depression, and other neuropsychiatric conditions. The German Study on the Epidemiology of Parkinson's disease (GEPAD) is a national representative epidemiological study of $n = 1{,}449$ PD patients, designed to estimate the prevalence of dementia, depression, and other neuropsychiatric conditions in PD patients of all stages [16]. Overall, next to depression with 33.6 % was dementia in 28.6 % of the patients, and additional clinically significant psychopathological syndromes in 61 %. Only 29.4 % had no neuropsychiatric conditions. This might explain the high rate of patients with depressive symptoms preoperatively (22 %) in our study. However, almost twice had, at least temporarily, depressive symptoms after the procedure. One explanation for this high rate might be that in the early years of DBS surgery, the medication was reduced very dramatically shortly after turning on the stimulation, a practice that has been abandoned due to these experiences. Appleby et al. found in their meta-analysis, contrary to our findings, an improvement in 83.3 % of studies reporting data on mood. Since a large number of studies did not report on post-DBS mood, the authors mentioned that this finding must be interpreted with caution.

There were no suicides (and no reported suicide attempts) in our patient group. Nevertheless, as mentioned previously, this risk has to be kept in mind, and patients have to be monitored carefully with regard to this topic pre- and postoperatively.

The high rate of preoperative comorbidity in patients with movement disorders, as well as the postoperative side-effects of DBS, stresses the need for a careful patient selection. Despite the high ratio of psychiatric symptoms in the post-

DBS course, most of the patients were very satisfied with the clinical result of DBS on the motor symptoms, and did not assess the overall effect of the DBS as negative. The vast majority (77 %) would choose to undergo the operation again due to the clinical benefit. Reasons for a negative retrospective attitude towards refusing surgery were in most cases poor motor improvement based on subjective judgement, or postoperative hardware complications. Only three patients (3.7 %) reported psychiatric AE after surgery as the reason for preferring to reject the surgery retrospectively.

Conclusion

A wide range of behavioural changes may be seen in patients eligible for deep brain surgery due to different kinds of movement disorders, as well as in the postoperative course. Depression and irritability were the most common side-effects after DBS in our study. PD patients, in contrast to dystonia and tremor patients, developed complications in all tested subgroups, with varying frequencies. Preoperative evaluation for psychiatric and cognitive dysfunction is crucial to identify patients who are at specific risk for psychiatric complications. Despite all these pitfalls, patients were overall very satisfied with the clinical result of the procedure, and would do it again in the vast majority of cases.

Conflict of Interest MOP, FA, GN received speaking honoraria from Medtronic.

References

1. Deuschl G, Schade-Brittinger C, Krack P, Volkmann J, Schafer H, Botzel K, Daniels C, Deutschlander A, Dillmann U, Eisner W, Gruber D, Hamel W, Herzog J, Hilker R, Klebe S, Kloss M, Koy J, Krause M, Kupsch A, Lorenz D, Lorenzl S, Mehdorn HM, Moringlane JR, Oertel W, Pinsker MO, Reichmann H, Reuss A, Schneider GH, Schnitzler A, Steude U, Sturm V, Timmermann L, Tronnier V, Trottenberg T, Wojtecki L, Wolf E, Poewe W, Voges J, German Parkinson Study Group, Neurostimulation Section (2006) A randomized trial for deep brain stimulation in Parkinson's disease. N Engl J Med 355:896–908
2. Weaver FM, Follett K, Stern M, CSP 468 Study Group et al (2009) Bilateral deep brain stimulation vs best medical therapy for patients with advanced Parkinson's disease: a randomized controlled trial. JAMA 301:63–73
3. Kupsch A, Benecke R, Muller J, Trottenberg T, Schneider GH, Poewe W, Eisner W, Wolters A, Muller JU, Deuschl G, Pinsker MO, Skogseid IM, Roeste GK, Vollmer-Haase J, Brentrup A, Krause M, Tronnier V, Schnitzler A, Voges J, Nikkhah G, Vesper J, Naumann M, Volkmann J, Deep-Brain Stimulation for Dystonia Study Group (2006) Pallidal deep-brain stimulation in primary generalized or segmental dystonia. N Engl J Med 355:1978–1990
4. Vidailet M, Vercueil L, Hueto JL, Krystkowiak P, Benabid AL, Cornu P, Lagrange C, Tezenas du Montcel S, Dormont D, Grand S, Blond S, Detante O, Pillon B, Ardouin C, Agid Y, Destee A, Pollak P, French Stimulation du Pallidum Interne dans la Dystonie (SPIDY) Study Group (2005) Bilateral deep-brain stimulation of the globus pallidus in primary generalized dystonia. N Engl J Med 352(5):459–467
5. Mehdorn HM, Goebel S, Falk D, Volkmann J, Leplow B, Pinsker MO (2008) Deep brain stimulation for movement disorders and its neuropsychological implications. Acta Neurochir 101:9–12
6. Funkiewiez A, Ardouin C, Caputo E, Krack P, Fraix V, Klinger H, Chabardes S, Foote K, Benabid AL, Pollak P (2004) Long term effects of bilateral subthalamic stimulation on cognitive function, mood, and behaviour in Parkinson's disease. J Neurol Neurosurg Psychiatry 75:834–839
7. Parsons TD, Rogers SA, Braaten AJ, Woods SP, Tröster AI (2006) Cognitive sequelae of subthalamic nucleus deep brain stimulation in Parkinson's disease: a meta-analysis. Lancet Neurol 5:578–588
8. Speelman JD, Smeding HM, Schmannd B (2007) Does chronic subthalamic nucleus stimulation in advanced Parkinson's disease cause invalidating cognitive and behavioural dysfunctions? J Neurol Neurosurg Psychiatry 78(3):221
9. Cummings JL, Mega M, Gray K, Rosenberg-Thompson S, Carusi DA, Gornbein J (1994) The Neuropsychiatric Inventory: comprehensive assessment of psychopathology in dementia. Neurol 44:2308–2314
10. Aarsland D, Cummings JL, Larsen JP (2001) Neuropsychiatric differences between Parkinson's disease with dementia and Alzheimer's disease. Int J Geriatr Psychiatry 16(2):184–191
11. Aarsland D, Brønnick K, Ehrt U, De Deyn PP, Tekin S, Emre M, Cummings JL (2007) Neuropsychiatric symptoms in patients with Parkinson's disease and dementia: frequency, profile and associated care giver stress. J Neurol Neurosurg Psychiatry 78(1): 36–42
12. Ferri CP, Prince M, Brayne C, Brodaty H, Fratiglioni L, Ganguli M, Hall K, Hasegawa K, Hendrie H, Huang Y, Jorm A, Mathers C, Menezes PR, Rimmer E, Scazufca M, and for the Alzheimer's Disease International (2005) Global prevalence of dementia: a Delphi consensus study. Lancet 366:2112–2117
13. Appleby BS, Duggan PS, Regenberg A, Rabins PV (2007) Psychiatric and neuropsychiatric adverse events associated with deep brain stimulation: a meta-analysis often years' experience. Mov Disord 22(12):1722–1728
14. Witt K, Daniels C, Reiff J, Krack P, Volkmann J, Pinsker MO, Krause M, Tronnier V, Kloss M, Schnitzler A, Wojtecki L, Bötzel K, Danek A, Hilker R, Sturm V, Kupsch A, Karner E, Deuschl G (2008) Neuropsychological and psychiatric changes after deep brain stimulation for Parkinson's disease: a randomised, multicentre study. Lancet Neurol 7:605–614
15. Daniels C, Krack P, Volkmann J, Pinsker MO, Krause M, Tronnier V, Kloss M, Schnitzler A, Wojtecki L, Bötzel K, Danek A, Hilker R, Sturm V, Kupsch A, Karner E, Deuschl G, Witt K (2010) Risk factors for executive dysfunction after subthalamic nucleus stimulation in Parkinson's disease. Mov Disord 25(11): 1583–1589
16. Von Reichmann H, Deuschl G, Riedel O, Spottke A, Förstl H, Henn F, Heuser I, Oertel W, Riederer P, Trenkwalder C, Dodel R, Wittchen HU (2010) The German study in the epidemiology of Parkinson's disease with dementia (GEPAD): more than Parkinson. MMW Fortschr Med 152(Suppl 1):1–6

Active Stimulation Site of Nucleus Accumbens Deep Brain Stimulation in Obsessive–Compulsive Disorder Is Localized in the Ventral Internal Capsule

Pepijn van den Munckhof, D. Andries Bosch, Mariska H.M. Mantione, Martijn Figee, Damiaan A.J.P. Denys, and P. Richard Schuurman

Abstract Obsessive–compulsive disorder (OCD) is a chronic psychiatric disorder characterized by persistent thoughts and repetitive ritualistic behaviours. Despite optimal cognitive–behavioral and pharmacological therapy, approximately 10 % of patients remain treatment-resistant. Deep brain stimulation (DBS) is being investigated as experimental therapy for treatment-refractory OCD. In the current study, we determined the relationship between anatomical location of active electrode contacts and clinical outcome in 16 OCD patients undergoing bilateral nucleus accumbens (NAc) DBS. We found that most patients actually do not receive active stimulation in the NAc but in the more laterally, anteriorly and dorsally located ventral part of the anterior limb of the internal capsule, ventral ALIC (vALIC). Our nine patients receiving bilateral vALIC DBS improved on average 73 % on their Yale-Brown Obsessive–Compulsive Scale (Y-BOCS) scores, whereas the six patients with their centers of stimulation located otherwise improved on average only 42 %. We therefore propose bilateral vALIC as a promising new DBS target for patients with treatment-refractory OCD. Future studies employing a direct vALIC targeting approach in larger patient numbers are needed to test whether this proposal holds true.

P. van den Munckhof (✉), D.A. Bosch, and P.R. Schuurman
Department of Neurosurgery H2-238,
Academic Medical Center, University of Amsterdam,
Meibergdreef 9, 1005 AZ Amsterdam, The Netherlands
e-mail: p.vandenmunckhof@amc.nl

M.H.M. Mantione, M. Figee, and D.A.J.P. Denys
Department of Psychiatry, Academic Medical Center,
University of Amsterdam, Meibergdreef 9,
1005 AZ Amsterdam, The Netherlands

Keywords Obsessive–compulsive disorder • Deep brain stimulation • Nucleus accumbens • Ventral part of the anterior limb of the internal capsule

Introduction

Obsessive–compulsive disorder (OCD) is a psychiatric disorder characterized by persistent thoughts (obsessions) and repetitive ritualistic behaviours (compulsions). Specific treatments for OCD have been developed, such as cognitive–behavioural therapy (CBT) and pharmacotherapy with serotonin reuptake inhibitors, but approximately 10 % of patients remain severely affected and suffer from treatment-refractory OCD [2]. There is evidence that deep brain stimulation (DBS) is effective in patients with treatment-refractory OCD when it is targeted at the anterior limb of the internal capsule (ALIC) [1, 16], subthalamic nucleus (STN) [13], ventral capsule/ventral striatum (VC/VS) [8], or nucleus accumbens (NAc) [3].

We recently reported 3–100 % decrease in obsessive–compulsive symptoms in 16 patients with treatment-refractory OCD undergoing bilateral implantation of small quadripolar DBS electrodes targeted at the NAc [3]. Interestingly, improvement was only observed when the upper two electrode contacts were used. The anatomical position of these two dorsal contacts theoretically varies between patients, depending on the sagittal and coronal angulations of electrode implantation. Some will be located towards the border between NAc and ventral part of the ALIC (vALIC), whereas others will be positioned more medially in the caudate nucleus (Cd), more laterally in the anterior part of the external globus pallidus (EGP), or more ventrally in the core of the NAc. In the current study, we determined the relationship between anatomical location of active electrode contacts and clinical outcome in these 16 patients with treatment-refractory OCD undergoing bilateral NAc DBS.

DOI 10.1007/978-3-7091-1482-7_9, © Springer-Verlag Wien 2013

Materials and Methods

Patients

Patients who received bilateral implantation of NAc DBS electrodes between April 2005 and December 2008 ($N=16$) were asked to participate in the current study to determine the relationship between anatomical location of active electrode contacts and long-term clinical outcome. Full details of inclusion and exclusion criteria have been described previously [3]. Briefly, patients were aged between 18 and 65 years, and were diagnosed with primary OCD according to criteria of the Diagnostic and Statistical Manual of Mental Disorders, fourth edition (DSM-IV), using the Structured Clinical Interview for DSM-IV Axis I disorders [4]. Only patients with a score of at least 28 on the Yale–Brown Obsessive Compulsive Scale (Y-BOCS) were included [6, 7]. Treatment-refractory was defined as no or insufficient response following at least two treatments with a selective serotonin reuptake inhibitor (SSRI) at maximum dose for at least 12 weeks, plus one treatment with clomipramine at maximum dose for at least 12 weeks with assessment of plasma levels to control for sufficient bioavailability, plus at least one augmentation trial with an atypical antipsychotic for 8 weeks in combination with an SSRI, plus at least one CBT trial for a minimum of 16 sessions. Patients with severe personality disorders and other clinically significant DSM-IV diagnoses were excluded, except for those with major depressive disorder and mild anxiety disorders. Other reasons for exclusion were clinically significant and unstable neurological or medical illnesses.

Surgical Procedure and Clinical Follow-Up

Implantation of the electrodes was performed with standard stereotactic procedures using frame-based 1.5 Tesla magnetic resonance imaging (MRI), with 1-mm slices for target determination. All 16 patients were implanted bilaterally with quadripolar electrodes (model 3389 Medtronic, Minneapolis, MN, USA), contact points being 1.5 mm long and separated from adjacent contacts by 0.5 mm. The contacts are coded from 0 (ventral) to 3 (dorsal), and are independently programmable. Target coordinates for electrode tips were 7 mm lateral to the midline, 3 mm anterior to the anterior border of the anterior commissure, and 4 mm inferior to the intercommissural line, in order to target the ventral contacts 0 and 1 in the NAc (according to the Atlas of the Human Brain by Mai et al. [12]). Electrodes were implanted with a sagittal angle of ±75° to the intercommissural line, and a coronal angle approximately following the ALIC into the NAc. Electrodes were connected via subcutaneous extensions to Soletra stimulators (Medtronic, Minneapolis) placed bilaterally in an infraclavicular pocket under general anesthesia. Correct stereotactic position of ventral electrode contact 0 was verified with postoperative stereotactic computer tomography (CT). After electrode implantation, patients were evaluated regularly for severity of symptoms and optimal stimulation parameters. Once an initial decrease in Y-BOCS score had been observed, which was on average after 8 weeks of stimulation, a standardized CBT program was added.

Clinical Outcome Measures

Obsessive–compulsive symptoms were measured with the Y-BOCS with scores ranging from 0 to 40; higher scores indicating more severe symptoms. A trained investigator completed the scales at baseline and on each follow-up visit.

Determination of Location of Active Electrode Contact

Since DBS electrodes may not have reached their final positions on immediate postoperative imaging [17], we analyzed anatomical locations of active electrode contacts on imaging after long-term follow-up, at least 11 months after electrode implantation. Patients underwent CT with 2 mm slices that was co-registered with the stereotactic planning MRI using Leksel Surgiplan® software (Elekta Instruments AB, Stockholm, Sweden). No clinical changes were observed during monopolar stimulation with case set positive and ventral contacts 0 and 1 set negative, and clinical improvement began only after switching to monopolar stimulation with dorsal contacts 2 and 3 negative [3]. The interspace between contact 2 and 3 (interspace 2/3), well-identifiable on CT (Fig. 1a), was therefore defined as the center of stimulation (Fig. 1b). For each patient, the anatomical location of the left- and right-sided center of stimulation was determined on the planning MRI and categorized to be in the NAc, more dorsally in vALIC, more medial in the Cd, more lateral in EGP or at the border between two of these structures (Fig. 1b). In addition, the lateral *X*, anterior-posterior *Y* and dorsal-ventral *Z* stereotactic distances in mm relative to the anterior border of the anterior commissure (AC) of each center of stimulation were calculated. The averaged left- and right-sided stereotactic centers of stimulation were calculated and projected into the *Stereotactic Atlas of the Human Thalamus and Basal Ganglia* by Morel [14].

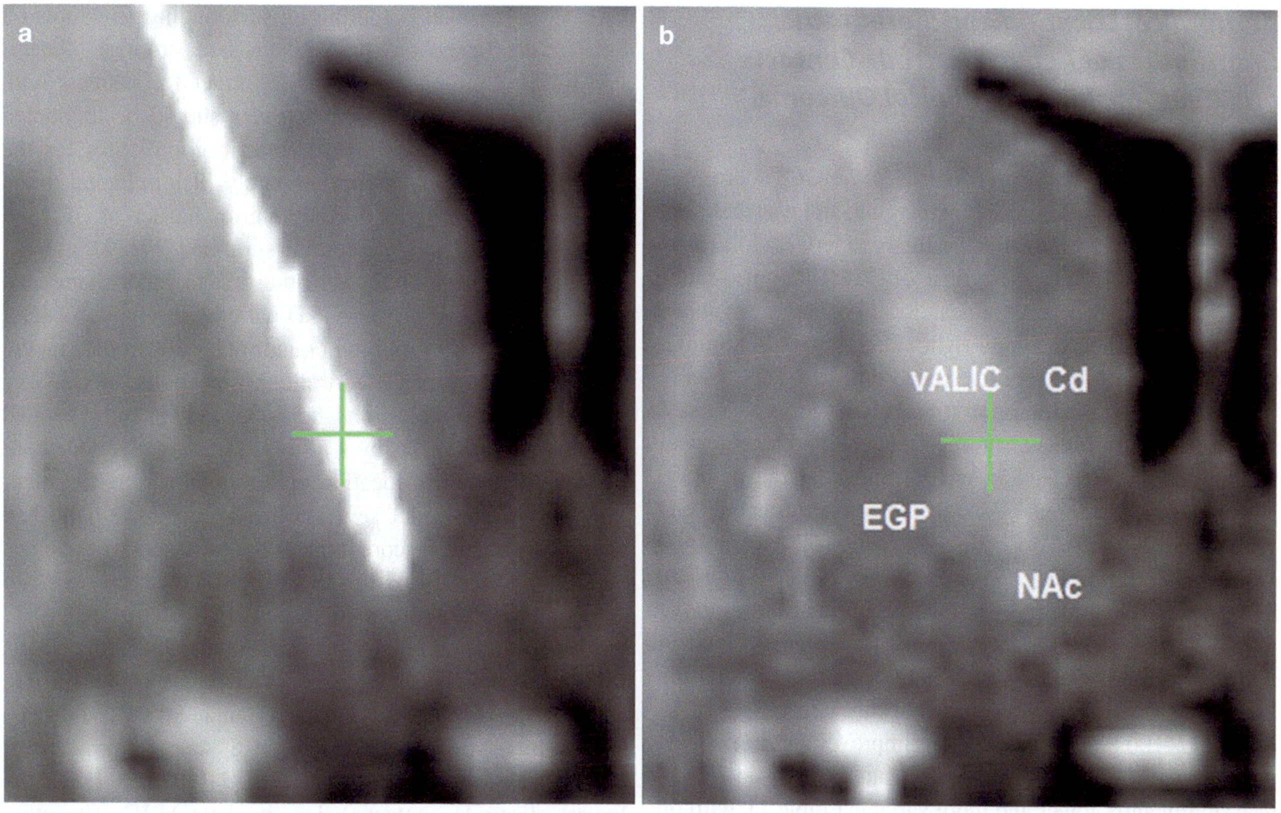

Fig. 1 Fused coronal images of stereotactic T1-weighted MRI and co-registered follow-up CT showing representative right-sided quadripolar electrode targeting the nucleus accumbens (NAc). The artefacts of the four individual electrode contacts are visible as separately distinguishable thickenings and interspace 2/3 is marked by the *green cross* (**a**). The neuro-anatomical location of interspace 2/3 can subsequently be categorized to be in the NAc, more dorsally in the ventral part of the anterior limb of the internal capsule (vALIC), more medially in the caudate nucleus (Cd), more laterally in the external globus pallidus (EGP) or at the border between two of these structures (**b**)

Statistical Analysis

Mean values are presented ± standard deviation. Y-BOCS scores were analyzed using paired *t*-test or Student's *t*-test. All statistical analyses were conducted with the SPSS statistical package version 16.0.

Results

Patient Characteristics, Stimulation Settings and Clinical Outcome

Mean age was 43 ± 11 years (range 26–59 years); six of the 16 patients were female, and mean follow-up was 50 ± 11 months (range 23–66 months). One patient fulfilled the DSM-IV criteria of obsessive–compulsive and avoidant personality disorder (pt 4). All patients started with monopolar stimulation with case positive and ventral contacts 0 and 1 set negative. Despite voltage increments, no patient reported clinical improvement. Improvement began only after switching to monopolar stimulation with dorsal contacts 2 and 3 set negative. Mean stimulation parameters were 4.7 ± 0.6 V (range 3.5–5.6 V), 103 ± 24 μs (range 90–150 μs) and 145 ± 25Hz (range 130–185 Hz). DBS resulted in a mean decrease of 19.8 ± 8.5 points (range 7–37 points) in Y-BOCS scores (60 %, $p<0.01$). Twelve patients (75 %) showed ≥35 % Y-BOCS score improvement, which is generally regarded as the definition of a responder to therapy in OCD literature. Responders and non-responders did not differ in demographic and clinical characteristics or stimulation parameters (data not shown), except for the content of the OCD symptoms; three non-responders (pts 4, 9 and 16) versus one responder (pt 10) suffered from egosyntonic obsessive–compulsive symptoms such as perfectionism, the need for symmetry, and hoarding. Responders had a mean decrease of 71 ± 19 % (range 45–100 %) on Y-BOCS scores versus 25 ± 5 % (range 22–32 %) decrease of Y-BOCS in non-responders.

Anatomical Location and Stereotactic Coordinates of Active Electrode Contacts and Relationship with Clinical Outcome

One patient (pt 1, 45 % improvement of Y-BOCS score) was not willing to undergo follow-up imaging, and was therefore excluded from analysis. Fifteen patients underwent follow-up CT, with a mean follow-up time of 36±9 months (range 11–52 months). The anatomical location and stereotactic coordinates of their left- and right-sided centers of stimulation are listed in Table 1, ordered according to Y-BOCS score improvement. The centers of stimulation were not located within the NAc (Table 1). In most patients, both centers of stimulation were located in vALIC, more lateral, anterior, and dorsal to the original NAc target, or at the border between vALIC and NAc or Cd (Table 1). When projected into the *Stereotactic Atlas of the Human Thalamus and Basal Ganglia* by Morel [14], the mean stereotactic coordinates of both the left- and right-sided center of stimulation were located in vALIC (Table 1). Patients with both centers of stimulation located in vALIC ($N=9$) improved on average 73±18 % (range 47–100 %). Y-BOCS score improvement in patients with their centers of stimulation located otherwise ($N=6$) was significantly lower and more variable (Table 1), with on average 42±28 % improvement (range 22–90 %, $p<0.05$). Among this latter group, two patients showed ≥35 % Y-BOCS score improvement (pts 7 and 15). Although both had their right-sided center of stimulation in vALIC or at the border between vALIC and NAc, this was also found in the four non-responders (Table 1). In three of the four non-responders, but only one of the responders, the left-sided center of stimulation was located in the more medially and anteriorly located Cd.

Discussion

In our series of 16 treatment-refractory OCD patients undergoing bilateral NAc DBS, obsessive–compulsive symptoms decreased by 60 % after a mean treatment period of 50 months, with 12 of 16 patients improving ≥35 % on Y-BOCS scores. Compared to our initial decrease of 52 % with nine of 16 patients responding after 21 months [3], these results show that DBS is an effective treatment for treatment-refractory OCD in the long term.

Analysis of anatomical locations of active electrode contacts showed that in most patients, the center of active stimulation was not in the NAc but in the more laterally, anteriorly, and dorsally located ventral part of the anterior limb of the internal capsule, vALIC. Best clinical results were obtained when both centers of active stimulation were located within vALIC, rather than bordering on surrounding structures on either side. Based on these results, we propose bilateral vALIC as a promising new DBS target for patients with treatment-refractory OCD: electrodes should be implanted following the ALIC, with stereotactic coordinates for the center of stimulation at approximately 11 mm lateral to the midline, 4 mm anterior to the anterior border of AC, and 3 mm superior to the intercommissural line (Fig. 2).

In 1999, Nuttin et al. were the first to report beneficial effects in three out of four OCD patients receiving bilateral ALIC DBS with 24 mm long quadripolar electrodes (model 3887 Pisces Compact, Medtronic, Minneapolis, MN, USA), with electrode contact points being 3 mm long and separated from adjacent contacts by 4 mm [15]. Active electrode contacts and anatomical location of stimulation were not mentioned. In recent years, several other groups have published significant Y-BOCS score improvements in series of patients undergoing bilateral ALIC DBS. Abelson et al. reported two responders out of four patients receiving bilateral ALIC DBS with 10.5 mm quadripolar electrodes (model 3387, Medtronic, Minneapolis), with electrode contact points being 1.5 mm long and separated from adjacent contacts by 1.5 mm [1]. The best responder (73 % Y-BOCS score improvement) received monopolar stimulation (7 V; 210 µs; 130 Hz) at the lowest electrode contact 0, i.e., in the vALIC. The other responder (44 % Y-BOCS score improvement) received bipolar stimulation (10.5 V; 210 µs; 130 Hz) using distal contacts 0, 1 and 2 as cathodes and proximal contact 3 as anode, which impedes pinpointing the center of active stimulation to a specific part of ALIC. Goodman et al. reported four responders (mean Y-BOCS score improvement of 62±20 %) out of six patients receiving bilateral ALIC DBS with 24-mm-long quadripolar electrodes (model 3887 Pisces Compact, Medtronic, Minneapolis), with electrode contact points being 3 mm long and separated from adjacent contacts by 4 mm and contact 0 in the region of the posterior border of AC [5]. In almost all patients, the center of clinically effective stimulation (4.6±2.4 V; 165±57 µs; 134±3 Hz) was located at the interspace between contact 0 and 1 or at contact 1, i.e., more laterally, anteriorly, and dorsally than the posterior border of AC. The largest series of patients was published by Greenberg et al., who reported 16 responders out of 26 patients receiving bilateral implantation of similarly large quadripolar electrodes targeting the ALIC [8]. When the implantation site of contact 0 was moved posteriorly (from 5 to 6 mm anterior of AC to 0 mm anterior of AC) towards the junction of the ALIC, AC, and bed nucleus of the stria terminalis (BST), more responders (from 33 to 75 %), larger mean Y-BOCS score improvements (from 29 to 54 %) and lower stimulation settings (from 8.4 V; 310 µs to 4.8 V; 185 µs) were noted. Most patients received monopolar stimulation at 'ventral contacts 0 and/or 1', but the exact anatomical sites of active stimulation were not mentioned.

Table 1 Stimulation settings, Y-BOCS score improvement, MRI location and stereotactic coordinates of left- and right-sided center of stimulation in OCD patients undergoing DBS targeted to the NAc, ordered according to Y-BOCS score improvement

Pt	Stim[a] V-µs-Hz	Y-BOCS improv (%)	MRI left	*X* left	*Y* left	*Z* left	MRI right	*X* right	*Y* right	*Z* right
14	5.6-150-130	28→0 (100 %)	vALIC	8.9	2.5	3.7	vALIC	12.5	2.9	3
11	3.5-90-130	38→1 (97 %)	vALIC	11.4	3.4	5	vALIC	9.9	6.3	5.9
7	5-90-130	30→3 (90 %)	EGP	13	4.2	2	vALIC/NAc	9.9	2.2	−1.1
5	4-90-185	33→5 (85 %)	vALIC	11.7	6.5	3.4	vALIC	11.8	6.1	3.3
12	5-90-185	33→10 (70 %)	vALIC	13.2	4.4	2.1	vALIC	13.5	3.9	2.7
8	5-90-130	35→9 (74 %)	vALIC	10.7	4	1	vALIC	10.2	3	1.5
13	4.5-90-185	35→11 (69 %)	vALIC	10.8	4.2	4.2	vALIC	10.7	3.8	1.8
15	4.5-90-130	29→11 (62 %)	Cd	11.7	4.7	0	vALIC	12.1	2.7	0.3
2	5.4-90-130	34→14 (59 %)	vALIC	11.4	3.4	2.1	vALIC	11.4	3.9	2.4
3	4.5-120-130	36→16 (56 %)	vALIC	9.2	4	2.1	vALIC	10.8	2.8	1.4
10	4.4-150-130	30→16 (47 %)	vALIC	10	4.9	3.7	vALIC	10.9	5.4	4.7
6	5.2-90-130	31→21 (32 %)	Cd	9.4	4.9	2.5	vALIC	10.5	3.3	1.3
9	5.5-90-185	38→29 (24 %)	vALIC/NAc	10.9	4.9	2.2	vALIC/NAc	11.3	4.3	1.5
4	3.7-90-130	40→31 (23 %)	Cd	10.3	4.7	1.6	vALIC	10.2	4.4	0.1
16	5-150-185	32→25 (22 %)	Cd	9.7	5.6	1.1	vALIC/NAc	11.6	3.6	0.7
Mean (SD)	4.7-104-148 (0.6-25-27)	33→13 (61 %)	vALIC[b]	10.8 (1.3)	4.4 (1.0)	2.4 (1.3)	vALIC[b]	11.1 (1.0)	3.9 (1.2)	2.0 (1.8)

Cd caudate nucleus, *DBS* deep brain stimulation, *EGP* external globus pallidus, *Hz* hertz, *Improv* improvement, *MRI* magnetic resonance imaging, *µs* microsecond, *NAc* nucleus accumbens, *OCD* obsessive–compulsive disorder, *Pt* patient inclusion number in original study (Denys et al. [3]), *Stim* stimulation parameters, *V* volt, *vALIC* ventral part of the anterior limb of the internal capsule, *Y-BOCS* Yale–Brown Obsessive Compulsive Scale

[a]All patients received monopolar stimulation with case positive and dorsal contacts 2 and 3 set negative

[b]According to *Stereotactic Atlas of the Human Thalamus and Basal Ganglia* by Morel [14]

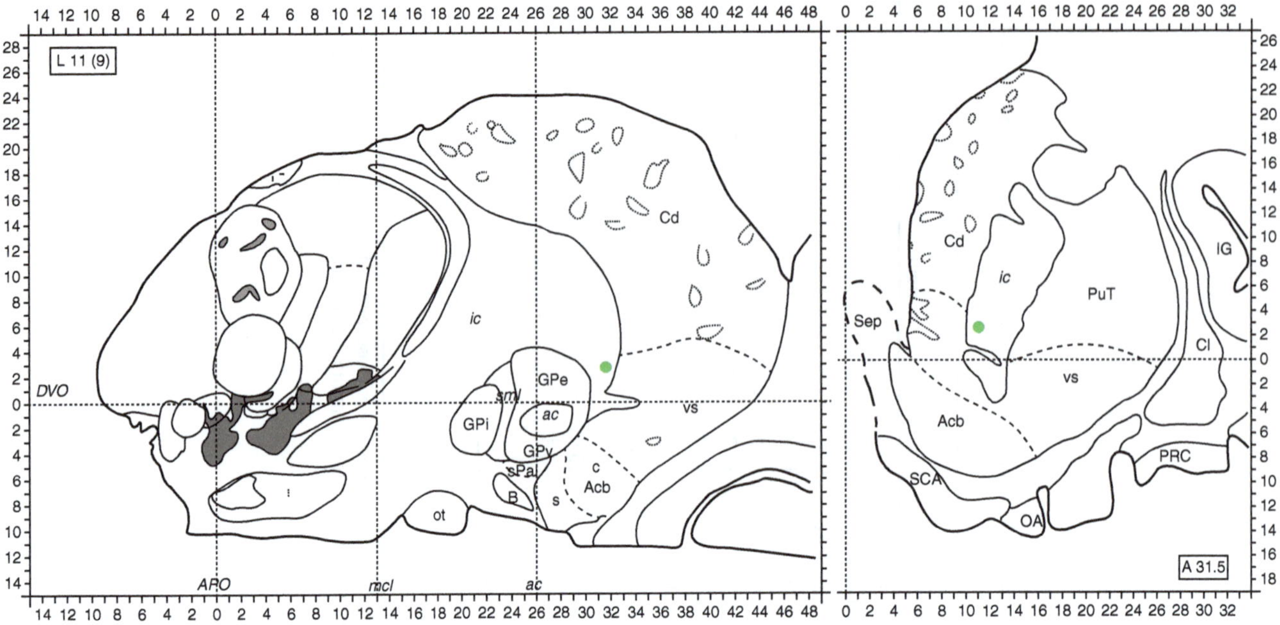

Fig. 2 Projection of vALIC DBS target for treatment-refractory OCD into sagittal plate L11 (*left panel*) and coronal plate A31.5 (*right panel*) of the *Stereotactic Atlas of the Human Thalamus and Basal Ganglia* [14]. Sagittal plate L11 corresponds with a sagittal plane located 11 mm lateral from the midline. Coronal plate A31.5 corresponds with a coronal plane located 4.5 mm anterior of the anterior border of AC. Stereotactic coordinates of vALIC are approximately 11 mm lateral to the midline, 4 mm anterior to the anterior border of AC, and 3 mm superior to the intercommissural line. Abbreviations: *ac* anterior commisure, *Acb* nucleus accumbens, *B* basal nucleus of Meynert, *c* Acb core, *Cd* caudate nucleus, *Cl* claustrum, *GPe* external globus pallidus, *GPi* internal globus pallidus, *GPv* ventral globus pallidus, *ic* internal capsule, *IG* insular gyrus, *iml* internal medullary lamina, *OA* olfactory area, *ot* optic tract, *PRC* piriform cortex, *PuT* putamen, *s* Acb shell, *SCA* subcallosal area, *Sep* septal area, *sPal* subpallidal area, *VS* ventral striatum

Can we determine the optimal DBS location for OCD? The mean Y-BOCS score improvement in our nine patients receiving bilateral vALIC DBS is very high, compared to previously published patients undergoing bilateral ALIC or bilateral STN DBS [13], suggesting that vALIC might be the brain target of choice for DBS in OCD. Active stimulation in the best responder from Abelson et al. was also bilaterally located in vALIC, albeit slightly more ventrally [1]. Electrode tips in patients from Goodman et al. and in the recently implanted patients from Greenberg et al. were located at a more medial, more posterior, and more ventral location than our vALIC target [5, 8]. But their larger electrode contact and interspace design, together with the fact that many of their patients received stimulation around contacts 0 and 1 or around contact 1, results in active stimulation at a more lateral, more anterior, and more dorsal location. This location might be very close to our currently proposed vALIC target.

The result of DBS in our series could, of course, not be solely determined by the anatomical location of stimulation. First, the addition of CBT was an important factor adding to the improvement in our patients [3], although this was applied to both patients with their active electrode contacts in vALIC and those with their active electrode contacts outside vALIC. Second, three out of the four non-responders (versus one out of 12 responders) suffered from egosyntonic OCD symptoms such as perfectionism, the need for symmetry, or hoarding. Perhaps, such egosyntonic content is a negative response predictor for DBS?

OCD is known to be associated with hyperactivity of cortical–striatal–pallidal–thalamic–cortical (CSTC) circuits connecting the orbitofrontal cortex (OFC), dorsal anterior cingulate cortex (dACC), ventromedial prefrontal cortex (vmPFC), caudate nucleus, NAc, pallidum, STN, and thalamus [9, 11]. The projections from the OFC, dACC, and vmPFC to the basal ganglia run through the ALIC [9, 10]. According to Greenberg et al., vALIC predominantly harbours CSTC fibers from OFC and vmPFC, whereas dorsal ALIC harbours fibers from dorsomedial PFC and dACC [9]. Based on our current findings, we hypothesize that modulation of hyperactive OFC and vmPFC fibers running through vALIC results in clinical improvement in treatment-refractory OCD patients receiving bilateral vALIC DBS. Indeed, Abelson et al. showed decreased OFC PET-activity following bilateral ALIC DBS in responders but not in non-responders [1]. We cannot rule out that part of our observed stimulation effects is due to spreading of current from vALIC to adjacent brain nuclei. However, the more medially located Cd seems an unlikely candidate, since three of four nonresponders had active left-sided stimulation in Cd. The more ventrally located NAc seems neither directly involved because none of our 16 patients reported improvement while employing monopolar stimulation with case positive and ventral contacts 0 and 1 set negative. On the other hand, spreading of current to the more laterally located EGP could in theory be involved, since our one patient with active left-sided stimulation in EGP improved 90 % on Y-BOCS score.

In summary, bilateral vALIC DBS seems highly effective in treatment-refractory OCD patients. Future studies employing a direct vALIC-targeting approach in larger patient numbers are needed to test whether this proposal holds true, and further neuroimaging studies in both responders and non-responders are needed to enlarge our understanding of this promising therapy.

Conflict of Interest The DBS devices used in the current patients were provided by Medtronic in the form of an unrestricted investigator-initiated research grant to Dr Denys and Dr Schuurman during the original study by Denys et al. [3]. The department of neurosurgery of the AMC has received an unrestricted grant for movement disorders research from Medtronic. Dr van den Munckhof has received travel grants from Medtronic. Dr Schuurman has received travel grants from Medtronic, and acts as independent advisor for Medtronic on educational matters. No other financial interest or potential conflicts are reported.

References

1. Abelson JL, Curtis GC, Sagher O, Albucher RC, Harrigan M, Taylor SF, Martis B, Giordani B (2005) Deep brain stimulation for refractory obsessive-compulsive disorder. Biol Psychiatry 57:510–516
2. Denys D (2006) Pharmacotherapy of obsessive-compulsive disorder and obsessive-compulsive spectrum disorders. Psychiatr Clin North Am 29:553–584
3. Denys D, Mantione M, Figee M, van den Munckhof P, Koerselman F, Westenberg H, Bosch DA, Schuurman PR (2010) Deep brain stimulation of the nucleus accumbens for treatment-refractory obsessive-compulsive disorder. Arch Gen Psychiatry 67:1061–1068
4. First MB, Spitzer RL, Gibbon MG, Williams JB (1997) Structured clinical interview for DSM-IV Axis I disorders (SCID-I): clinical version. American Psychiatric Press, Washington, D.C
5. Goodman WK, Foote KD, Greenberg BD, Ricciuti N, Bauer R, Ward H, Shapira NA, Wu SS, Hill CL, Rasmussen SA, Okun MS (2010) Deep brain stimulation for intractable obsessive compulsive disorder: pilot study using a blinded staggered-onset design. Biol Psychiatry 67:535–542
6. Goodman WK, Price LH, Rasmussen SA, Mazure C, Delgado P, Heninger GR, Charney DS (1989) The Yale-Brown Obsessive Compulsive Scale, II: validity. Arch Gen Psychiatry 46:1012–1016
7. Goodman WK, Price LH, Rasmussen SA, Mazure C, Fleischmann RL, Hill CL, Heninger GR, Charney DS (1989) The Yale-Brown Obsessive Compulsive Scale, I: development, use, and reliability. Arch Gen Psychiatry 46:1006–1011
8. Greenberg BD, Gabriels LA, Malone DA Jr, Rezai AR, Friehs GM, Okun MS, Shapira NA, Foote KD, Cosyns PR, Kubu CS, Malloy PF, Salloway SP, Giftakis JE, Rise MT, Machado AG, Baker KB, Stypulkowski PH, Goodman WK, Rasmussen SA, Nuttin BJ (2010) Deep brain stimulation of the ventral internal capsule/ventral striatum for obsessive-compulsive disorder: worldwide experience. Mol Psychiatry 15:64–79
9. Greenberg BD, Rauch SL, Haber SN (2010) Invasive circuitry-based neurotherapeutics: stereotactic ablation and deep brain stimulation for OCD. Neuropsychopharamcology 35:317–336
10. Gutman DA, Holtzheimer PE, Behrens TEJ, Johansen-Beerg H, Mayberg HS (2009) A tractography analysis of two deep brain stimulation white matter targets for depression. Biol Psychiatry 65:276–282
11. Haynes WIA, Mallet L (2010) High-frequency stimulation of deep brain structures in obsessive-compulsive disorders: the search for a valid circuit. Eur J Neurosci 32:1118–1127
12. Mai JK, Assheuer J, Paxinos G (1997) Atlas of the human brain. Academic, San Diego
13. Mallet L, Polosan M, Jaafari N, Baup N, Welter ML, Fontaine O, du Montcel ST, Yelnik J, Chéreau I, Arbus C, Raoul S, Aouizerate B, Damier P, Chabardès S, Czernecki V, Ardouin C, Krebs MO, Bardinet E, Chaynes P, Burbaud P, Cornu P, Derost P, Bougerol T, Bataille B, Mattei V, Dormont D, Devaux B, Vérin M, Houeto JL, Pollak P, Benabid AL, Agid Y, Krack P, Millet B, Pelissolo A, STOC Study Group (2008) Subthalamic nucleus stimulation in severe obsessive-compulsive disorder. N Engl J Med 359:2121–2134
14. Morel A (2007) Stereotactic atlas of the human thalamus and basal ganglia. Informa Healthcare, New York
15. Nuttin B, Cosyns P, Demeulemeester H, Gybels J, Meyerson B (1999) Electrical stimulation in anterior limbs of internal capsules in patients with obsessive-compulsive disorder. Lancet 354:1526
16. Nuttin BJ, Gabriëls LA, Cosyns PR, Meyerson BA, Andréewitch S, Sunaert SG, Maes AF, Dupont PJ, Gybels JM, Gielen F, Demeulemeester HG (2003) Long-term electrical capsular stimulation in patients with obsessive-compulsive disorder. Neurosurgery 52:1263–1272
17. Van den Munckhof P, Contarino MF, Bour LJ, Speelman JD, de Bie RMA, Schuurman PR (2010) Postoperative curving and upward displacement of deep brain stimulation electrodes caused by brain shift. Neurosurgery 67:49–54

Functional Neurosurgery for Secondary Dystonia: Indications and Long-Term Results

Jairo Alberto Espinoza Martinez, Oscar Andres Escobar Vidarte, and Gabriel Arango Uribe

Abstract Dystonia is a movement disorder characterized by patterned, repetitive, phasic, or tonic sustained muscle contractions that produce abnormal, often twisting, postures or repetitive movements. When the disorder is genetic or the cause is unknown and dystonia is the sole feature, the disease is called primary or idiopathic, conversely secondary dystonia (SD) may be caused by various brain insults. Both primary dystonia and SD have been notorious for their poor response to medical treatment. Today, stereotactic neurosurgical procedures are offered to improve the disability and quality of life of patients who do not respond to medical therapy. However, SD shows less and more variable results than primary dystonia to neurosurgical procedures, the benefits of ablative or deep brain stimulation (DBS) procedures in basal structures being still subject to debate and much harder to fully appreciate. In this work, the authors show a 33-patient series with secondary dystonia, separating the statistic and clinical analysis into several etiology groups: perinatal insults, tardive syndromes, genetic syndromes, and posttraumatic. In these groups, we show the mean BFM score improvement in the different patient series, comparing our results with world literature, and finally propose a classification system for bettering the clinical approach in surgery decision when this is indicated.

Keywords Secondary dystonia • Deep brain stimulation • Intrathecal baclofen • Brain motor circuits

J.A.E. Martinez (✉), O.A.E. Vidarte, and G.A. Uribe
Movement Disorders and Pain Management Center, CIMAD, Calle 19 A # 82-14, Bogota, Colombia

Marly Clinic, Bogota, Colombia

San Jose Children's Hospital, Bogota, Colombia
e-mail: jairoespinoza@cimad.net.co; neuroescobar@yahoo.com; gjarango@gmail.com

Introduction

Dystonia is a movement disorder characterized by patterned, repetitive, phasic, or tonic sustained muscle contractions that produce abnormal, often twisting, postures or repetitive movements [1, 2]. When the disorder is genetic or the cause is unknown and dystonia is the sole feature, the disease is called primary or idiopathic; conversely, secondary dystonia (SD) may be caused by various brain insults [2, 3] (Table 1).

Both primary (especially generalized) and SD have been notorious for their poor response to medical treatment; stereotactic functional neurosurgical procedures are offered to improve the disability and quality of life of patients who do not respond to medical therapy. Nowadays, the preferred surgical target in primary dystonia patients is the globus pallidus internus (Gpi) [1, 2, 4–13], with encouraging results reported in the long term. In contrast to the overall good response in patients with idiopathic dystonia, patients with SD showed less and more variable results with functional neurosurgical brain Gpi procedures, the benefit of deep brain stimulation (DBS) in this target for SD being still subject to debate and much harder to fully appreciate [1, 2, 12, 13]. In this chapter, we show our surgical experience in secondary dystonia and our proposal to separate disease entities to a better systematic approach in these patients.

Materials and Methods

Ninety patients were submitted to our unit with the diagnosis of secondary dystonia to consider functional neurosurgery. All of them had a request for deep brain stimulation. All cases were thoroughly studied by our interdisciplinary Movement Disorders Team, and medically treated before surgery when necessary.

Fifteen patients were ruled out because of very poor clinical condition, mild disease not impacting on quality of life, or

G. Nikkhah and M. Pinsker (eds.), *Stereotactic and Functional Neurosurgery*, Acta Neurochirurgica Supplement, Vol. 117,
DOI 10.1007/978-3-7091-1482-7_10, © Springer-Verlag Wien 2013

Table 1 Characteristics that suggest secondary dystonia diagnosis

Characteristics that suggest secondary dystonia diagnosis
History of possible etiology (traumatic brain injury, trauma peripheral perinatal noxa, encephalitis, toxic exposure or medications, encephalitis)
Neurological abnormality other than dystonia present
Examination findings suggest psychogenic origin
Dystonia is present at rest, rather than on action
Site of initiation and progression does not correspond to a known pattern of primary dystonia
Hemidystonia
Abnormal brain imaging
Abnormal laboratory findings suggesting any etiology

not fulfilling inclusion criteria. Seventy-five were operated either with DBS, intrathecal baclofen (ITB), or both. Forty-two of them were diagnosed as primary dystonia, and are excluded from this analysis, whereas 33 were operated because of some form of SD (Table 2). The SD group was followed up; we compared the Burke–Fahn–Marsden (BFM) dystonia rating scores and subjective scores before and after surgery, to establish mean improvement.

Results

The patients were separated into four broad categories according to the suspected or diagnosed etiology: SD to perinatal insults, tardive syndromes (TS), genetic syndromes and posttraumatic cases. This 33-patient series had a total mean BFM improvement of *41.6 %* (Tables 3).

SD Perinatal Insults: This group consists of 21 cases followed up for a period of 6 to up to 120 months; four ITB pumps and 17 Gpi DBS systems were implanted (Table 2). In patients with pure dystonia (without spasticity), there was a mean improvement of *43.4 %* in the BFM score after Gpi DBS (Table 3). The improvement was greater in the generalized early-onset secondary dystonia (G EOSD) and hemidystonia groups, with *41.8 %* and *75.8 %* of improvement in BFM score (not including patients with spasticity) (Table 3). Among patients with cerebral palsy, the maximal benefit occurred in one patient with the dyskinetic type operated with Gpi DBS, showing a reduction of *61.2 %* in BFM score. Patients of the mixed type of CP achieved a mean improvement of *20.3 %* (DBS) and *38.7 %* (ITB) (gross total CP group improvement in BFM score of *27.2 %*) (Table 3). Among Gpi DBS patients, there were two cases not having meaningful improvement which required ITB pump implantation. These two cases showed a synergistic therapeutic improvement, leading to *48.6 %* of improvement in BFM score after both systems were programmed. Encouraged by these results, we have indicated ITB pumps in previously Gpi DBS operated patients who no longer benefited from the latter surgery, or in those whose benefit was rather small (cases MV, FS, WS and RG) and the added benefit has averaged 50 %. ITB pumps benefited all mixed type of CP (M CP) patients in terms of having less pain, spasticity, or dyskinetic movements. Whereas patients and parents or caregivers were satisfied by the results, BFM scores dropped by *38.7 %* on average and Ashworth scores decreased at least by 50 %.

Tardive Syndromes: TS consisted of eight cases followed up for a period of 6 months up to 78 months. All cases were exposed to psychiatric medications because of psychiatric diseases (paranoid schizophrenia, bipolar disorder, major depression, anxiety), drug addictions, and in one case, medication was self-prescribed to alleviate insomnia. Patients used typical antipsychotics for more than 6 months, the most frequent being haloperidol and levomepromazine. All labs and neuroimaging studies were normal. All patients were diagnosed as having tardive dystonia as the dominant movement disorder; not infrequently, these patients showed features of a tardive dyskinetic syndrome, which was focalized in the orofacial region. SD was distributed in a segmental (S TS) pattern in six cases, and was generalized (G TS) in two. The BFM score improved in all cases after Gpi DBS, *72.6 %* being the mean reduction in this score (Table 3). The mean change in G TS was *70.6* and *73.4 %* in S TS (Table 3). Complications appeared in two cases. The case NT was surgically revised because extension cables broke 1 month after surgery. The cause was violent movements that subjected the cables to shearing forces. Patient LM had extreme cachexia with a very thin skin. Erosions around frontal incisions and pectoral area ensued in this female patient, and therefore surgical revision was needed. Overall, patients rated the results as excellent, and were all satisfied, despite the mean improvement on the scales. Interestingly, patients AL and NT were not responding adequately to antipsychotic medications for their psychiatric pathologies, and after months of continuous DBS their response rate increased. Dosage was not altered, and they appeared to be in remission (schizophrenia and bipolar disorder respectively) on the long-term follow-up.

Genetic Syndromes: The group consisted of three cases followed up for a period of 9 months up to 36 months. All cases were studied and diagnosed with genetic syndromes by movement disorders specialists: dystonia-parkinsonism, pantothenate kinase-associated neurodegeneration and secondary degenerative dystonia (Wilson's disease). MRI in the first case was normal (GL); the second patient (SC) showed the typical bilateral eye of the tiger sign in the T2 weighted sequences, whereas the third case (RG) showed increased copper and ceruloplasmine levels. After Gpi DBS, GL achieved an improvement of *55.6 %* in BFM score (Table 3); especially in tonic component and parkinsonism-related ON medication, dyskinesias almost disappeared. SC had generalized signs, with painful and tonic contractions dominating the clinical picture; after ITB pump implantation, the patient

Table 2 Clinical characteristics in a 33-patient series with secondary dystonia

Case	Age	Laboratories	Neuro-imaging	Previous diseases	Diagnosis	Surgery
EW	14	N	N	Perinatal hypoxia?	G EOSD	DBS Gpi B
SM	14	N	Mild generalized brain atrophy	Perinatal hypoxia	M CP	Baclofen pump
YP	23	N	Mild cortical and caudate atrophy, more right	Perinatal hypoxia	D CP	DBS Gpi B
JS	16	N	Mild generalized brain atrophy	Perinatal hypoxia	G EOSD	DBS Gpi B
YL	17	N	Chiari I malformation	Perinatal hypoxia?	Hemidystonia	DBS Gpi B
IC	10	N	Small left occipital atrophic area	Perinatal hypoxia?	G EOSD	DBS Gpi B
MV	15	N	Mild generalized brain atrophy	Kernicterus	M CP	DBS Gpi B
FS	27	N	Mild generalized brain atrophy	Perinatal hypoxia	M CP	DBS Gpi B
JM	28	N	N	Perinatal hypoxia	M CP	DBS Gpi B
YG	14	N	N	Perinatal hypoxia	M CP	Baclofen pump
AG	26	N	N	Perinatal hypoxia	M CP	DBS Gpi B
JA	8	N	N	No	M CP	Baclofen pump
GR	24	N	Bilateral Gpi, hyperintensities on MRI	Perinatal hypoxia	G EOSD	DBS Gpi B
WS	15	Slight increase in ceruloplasmine	N	Perinatal hypoxia	G EOSD	DBS Gpi B
RG	27	N	N	No	G EOSD	DBS Gpi B
AC	13	N	Small left temporo-mesial arachnoid cyst	Perinatal hypoxia	M CP	Baclofen pump
MC	36	N	N	No	Hemidystonia	DBS Gpi left
JA	27	N	N	No	G EOSD	DBS Gpi B
JP	16	N	N	Kernicterus	G EOSD	DBS Gpi B
JB	20	N	Mild generalized brain atrophy	Kernicterus	M CP	DBS Gpi B
JP	18	N	Left fronto-parietal cortical encephalomalacia	No	Hemidystonia	DBS Gpi I
NT	48	N	N	Psychiatric treatment	G TS	DBS Gpi B
JC	82	N	N	Psychiatric treatment	S TS	DBS Gpi B
CC	69	N	N	Psychiatric treatment	S TS	DBS Gpi B
EM	33	N	N	Self prescribed medications for insomnia	S TS	DBS Gpi B
IA	38	N	N	Psychiatric treatment	S TS	DBS Gpi B
LM	54	N	N	Psychiatric treatment	S TS	DBS Gpi B
ON	26	N	N	Multiple drug addictions	S TS	DBS Gpi B
AL	49	N	N	Multiple drug addictions	G EOSD	DBS Gpi B
GL	49	N	N	No	Parkinsonism dystonia	DBS Gpi B
SC	21	N	Bilateral eye of the tiger sign	No	Pantothenate kinase-associated neurodegeneration	Baclofen pump
RG	27	Increased copper and ceruloplasmine levels	Small sized basal ganglia nuclei	No	Secondary degenerative dystonia	DBS Gpi B
JT	47	N	N	Vehicle accident and prolonged coma	G LOSD	DBS Gpi L and R Pallidotomy

N normal, *G EOSD* generalized early onset secondary dystonia, *G LOSD* generalized late onset secondary dystonia, *M CP* mixed cerebral palsy, *D CP* dystonic cerebral palsy, *S TS* segmental tardive syndrome, *G TS* generalized tardive syndrome, *DBS Gpi* deep brain stimulation of globus pallidus internus

Table 3 Pre and post-operative Burke–Fahn–Marsden Scale in a 33-patient series with secondary dystonia

Case	Diagnosis	Surgery	Burke–Fahn–Marsden pre	Burke–Fahn–Marsden post
EW	G EOSD	DBS B Gpi	48 (3 – 3 – 12 – 2 – 6 – 6 – 8 – 4 – 4)	12 (0 – 0 – 8 – 0 – 1 – 1 – 1 – 0 – 1)
SM	M CP	Baclofen pump	76 (0 – 0 – 12 – 12 – 16 – 12 – 12 – 12 – 0). Ashworth 4.	32 (0 – 0 – 8 – 4 – 12 – 3 – 2 – 2 – 1). Ashworth 2 – 3
YP	D CP	DBS Gpi B	72 (0 – 8 – 12 – 8 – 16 – 16 – 3 – 3 – 6)	28 (0 – 0.5 – 8 – 1.5 – 3 – 3 – 3 – 3 – 6)
JS	G EOSD	DBS Gpi B	17 (0 – 0 – 0 – 8 – 4.5 – 4.5 – 0 – 0 – 0)	12.5 (0.5 – 0 – 0 – 3 – 0 – 0 – 0 – 0 – 9)
YL	Hemidystonia	DBS Gpi B	44 (0 – 3 – 1 – 8 – 16 – 0 – 0 – 0 – 16)	2 (0 – 0 – 1 – 1 – 0 – 0 – 0 – 0 – 0)
IC	G EOSD	DBS Gpi B	100.5 (0 – 0 – 16 – 4.5 – 16 – 16 – 16 – 16 – 16)	9 (0 – 0 – 4 – 0 – 1 – 1 – 1 – 1 –1)
MV	M CP	DBS Gpi B	78.5 (3 – 3 – 0 – 4.5 – 12 – 12 – 16 – 16 – 12)	65 (1.5 – 3 – 0 – 4.5 – 12 – 12 – 16 – 16 – 0)
FS	M CP	DBS Gpi B	87.5 (3 – 3 – 1 – 4.5 – 16 – 12 – 16 – 16 – 16). Ashworth 4	87.5 (3 – 3 – 1 – 4.5 – 16 – 12 – 16 – 16 – 16). Ashworth 4
JM	M CP	DBS Gpi B	44.5 (3 – 0 – 0 – 4.5 – 9 – 12 – 0 – 0 – 16)	18 (1.5 – 0 – 1 – 1.5 –6 – 6 – 0 – 0 – 2)
YG	M CP	Baclofen pump	77.5 (0 – 1.5 – 16 – 8 – 16 – 16 – 2 – 2 – 16). Ashworth 4.	60.5 (0 – 1.5 – 16 – 6 – 16 – 16 – 2 – 2 – 1). Ashworth 2 – 3
AG	M CP	DBS Gpi B	70.5 (1.5 – 8 – 9 – 12 – 16 – 16 – 0 – 0 – 8)	48.5 (1.5 – 8 – 9 – 6 – 9 – 9 – 0 – 0 – 6)
JA	M CP	Baclofen pump	93.5 (3 – 0.5 – 8 – 8 – 16 – 16 – 16 – 16 – 10). Ashworth 4	41 (1.5 – 0 – 8 – 1.5 – 8 – 9 – 2 – 2 – 9). Ashworth 2
GR	G EOSD	DBS Gpi B	64.5 (6 – 1.5 – 9 – 8 – 12 – 10 – 3 – 3 – 12)	34 (1.5 – 1.5 – 6 – 3 – 6 – 6 – 3 – 1 – 6)
WS	G EOSD	DBS Gpi B	61 (6 – 4 – 12 – 12 – 12 – 9 – 2 – 0 – 4)	59 (3 – 6 – 12 – 9 – 9 – 9 – 2 – 6 – 3)
RG	G EOSD	DBS Gpi B	120 (8 – 8 – 12 – 16 – 12 – 16 – 16 – 16 – 16)	116 (8 – 8 – 12 – 12 – 12 – 16 – 16 – 16 – 16)
AC	M CP	Baclofen pump	98.5 (3 – 2 – 16 – 1.5 – 16 – 16 – 16 – 16 – 12). Ashworth 4	81 (2 – 1.5 – 12 – 1.5 – 12– 12– 16 – 16 – 8). Ashworth 2
MC	Hemidystonia	DBS Gpi left	32 (0 – 0 – 0 – 0 – 16 – 0 – 0 – 16 – 0)	20 (0 – 0 – 0 – 0 – 12– 0 – 0 – 8 – 0). Mayor impacto en el caminar
JA	G EOSD	DBS Gpi B	94 (4.5 – 4.5 – 1 – 12 – 12 – 16 – 16 – 16 – 12)	40 (1.5 – 0 – 6 – 1.5 – 7 – 9 – 3 – 3 – 9)
JP	G EOSD	DBS Gpi B	86 (6 – 8 – 16 – 8 – 16 – 16 – 0 – 0 – 16)	62 (6 – 8 – 16 – 6 – 7 – 7 – 0 – 0 – 12)
JB	M CP	DBS Gpi B	69.5 (0.5 – 3 – 16 – 6 – 12 – 16 – 0 – 0 – 16)	60.5 (0.5 – 3 – 16 – 4 – 9 – 16 – 0 – 0 – 12)
JP	Hemidystonia	DBS Gpi I	48 (0 – 0 – 0 – 8 – 12– 0 – 12 – 0 – 16)	8 (0 – 0 – 0 – 0 – 3 – 0 – 3 – 0 – 2)
ON	S TS	DBS Gpi B	14.5 (0.5 – 1 – 1 – 8 – 2 – 1 – 0 – 0 – 1)	4 (0 – 0 – 0 – 3 – 0 – 0 – 0 – 0 – 1)
AL	G EOSD	DBS Gpi B	43 (3 – 3 – 1 – 3 – 16 – 16 – 0 – 0 – 1)	9 (1.5 – 1.5 – 0.5 – 0.5 – 1 – 1 – 0 – 0 – 3)
NT	G TS	DBS Gpi B	47 (6 – 8 – 6 – 8 – 2 – 1 – 0 – 0 – 16)	17.5 (4 – 4 – 3 – 1.5 – 1 – 1 – 0 – 0 – 3)
JC	S TS	DBS Gpi B	40 (8 – 8 – 12 – 6 – 0 – 0 – 0 – 0 – 6)	15 (4.5 – 1.5 – 3 – 3 – 0 – 0 – 0 – 0 – 3)
CC	S TS	DBS Gpi B	35 (8 – 8 – 6 – 12 – 1 – 0 – 0 – 0 – 0)	8 (1 – 1 – 3 – 2 – 1 – 0 – 0 – 0 – 0)
EM	S TS	DBS Gpi B	58 (6 – 3 – 1 – 8 – 4 – 4 – 8 – 8 – 16)	7.5 (0 – 3 – 1 – 0.5 – 1 – 1 – 0 – 0 – 1)
IA	S TS	DBS Gpi B	34 (8 – 6 – 12 – 6 – 0– 0 – 0 – 0 – 2)	16.5 (3 – 4.5 – 4 – 4 – 0 – 0 – 0 – 0 – 1)
LM	S TS	DBS Gpi B	36 (8 – 8 – 6 – 8 – 0 – 0 – 0 – 0 – 6)	7 (2 – 2 – 2 – 0.5 – 0 – 0 – 0 – 0 – 0.5)
GL	Parkinsonism dystonia	DBS Gpi B	9 (0 – 0 – 0 – 8 – 0 – 0 – 0 – 0 – 1)	4 (0 – 0 – 0 – 4 – 0 – 0 – 0 – 0 – 0)
SC	Pantothenate kinase-associated neurodegeneration	Baclofen pump	95.5 (6 – 0.5 – 9 – 8 – 16 – 16 – 12 – 12 – 16). Ashworth 4	60.5 (1 – 0.5 – 9 – 4 – 9 – 9 – 8 – 8 – 12). Ashworth 2 – 3
RG	Secondary degenerative dystonia	DBS Gpi B	120 (8 – 8 – 12 – 16 – 12 – 16 – 16 – 16 – 16)	116 (8 – 8 – 12 – 12 – 12 – 16 – 16 – 16 – 16)
JT	G LOSD	DBS Gpi I	64.5 (6 – 4.5 – 12 – 6 – 12– 12 – 0 – 0 – 12)	52.5 (6 – 4.5 – 12 – 3 – 9 – 9 – 0 – 0 – 9)

N normal, *G EOSD* generalized early onset secondary dystonia, *G LOSD* generalized late onset secondary dystonia, *M CP* mixed cerebral palsy, *D CP* dystonic cerebral palsy, *S TS* segmental tardive syndrome, *G TS* generalized tardive syndrome, *DBS Gpi* deep brain stimulation of globus pallidus internus

achieved a spasticity improvement of 50 %, thus facilitating daily care, and BFM scores dropped by *36.7 %* at the expense of reducing fixed postures (Table 3). RG had generalized signs as well, with painful and tonic axial and appendicular contractions, severely aggravated by stress. Grasping and manual functions were lost. A prominent arousal effect was evident each time the patient had a sensorial stimulus, then semi-ballistic movements appeared. Gpi DBS decreased this sign, while dystonia itself did not change significantly (*3.4 %* improvement in BFM score) (Table 3).

Posttraumatic: There was only one patient operated in this group, a 47-year-old male that suffered politrauma and severe head trauma with coma, needing prolonged intensive care. Brain MRI showed alterations compatible with diffuse axonal injury. After slow recovery, severe dysarthria and axial dystonia appeared. SD affected the superior extremities as well, leading to lost hand function. Surprisingly, neuropsychological evaluation showed little cognitive dysfunction. The patient firstly received a right pallidotomy, and 6 months afterwards left Gpi DBS. After pulse generator programming, the biggest improvement was seen on manual function (*25 %* improvement). Axial dystonia also decreased by *25 %*, and there was an improvement in BFM score of *18.7 %* (Table 3). The patient rates the result as satisfactory, because of pain and tonic SD reduction which had limited function and gate.

Discussion

SD is an entity where almost all syndromes not classifiable as primary are put together. Since the clinical expression of dystonia is very variable, as its multiple etiologies are, response to treatments and outcomes vary widely as well. Treatments offered to one type may be absolutely not helpful to other cases. A literature review shows that, in contrast to the overall good response with functional surgery in patients with idiopathic dystonia, patients with SD showed less and more variable benefit [1, 2, 5, 12, 13, 16–19]. The dystonia–choreoathetosis group secondary to cerebral palsy (CP) has shown variable mean improvements in BFM score with DBS [15, 24–26]; however, hemidystonia and TS groups have shown encouraging mean improvements in BFM scores in the long-term analysis [14, 20–23, 27, 28]. Finally, with regard to ITB therapy, this has been indicated in patients with SD, especially to CP, with the aim of reducing painful contractions, improve posture, and facilitate patient management by caregivers [29–31]; however, it also has been used in adult secondary dystonia [32, 33], with disappointing results reported by some [33, 34] and important anti-dystonic effects in the long-term analysis reported by others [30, 31, 35–42], with continuous improvement in comfort, mood, and quality of life of patients.

The authors feel it is necessary to find an alternative classification and grading system that will take into account the fact that SD encompasses diseases which are as different as their names are. A new classification system should bear in mind the fact that these diseases deserve different study approaches and treatments. As long as treatment response to brain procedures is different if brain circuitry is intact or not, and based on literature review and our experience, which is partially reported in this paper, we separate SD into two main types, as follows:

1. *Brain motor circuits intact*: in this group, diseases have not damaged the anatomy in such a significant way as to be demonstrable in neuroimaging. To this group belong patients with TS and some with perinatal insults (non-CP patients) and genetic syndromes. Hemidystonic patients have been included if there is no overt or gross abnormality in the basal ganglia.
2. *Brain motor circuits not intact*: here, posttraumatic and CP cases are included, and genetic or hemidystonic forms where significant anatomical alterations are seen in the basal ganglia.

The importance of separating the SD forms is that treatments could be offered to patients with a reasonable degree of success. Patients with normal anatomy should benefit from DBS as the first alternative, whereas patients with altered anatomy should be divided into groups to decide between DBS or ITB at this time:

1. *Hemidystonia group*: they should receive a DBS trial.
2. *CP group*: ITB trial should be the first step. Since published literature shows conflicting results, and our group is too small to draw firm conclusions, we offer patients a trial using progressively higher doses of baclofen first. Titrating doses to up to 150 mcg, we have seen responses in patients previously declared as not candidates with 100 mcg.

In patients not responding to the ITB trial, a DBS trial is offered. Gpi is our first target when tonic component predominates. In cases with dystonic tremor or not responding to Gpi DBS, we propose Vim (Ventralis Intermedius nucleus), Vop (Ventralis Oralis Posterior nucleus) or subthalamic DBS. There are ongoing trials using cortical or other deep targets and the internal capsule, targets with which we have no experience. They could be tried in selected cases. About posttraumatic dystonia, no recommendations can be made out of a single case, except that, based on this case and mostly on the literature review, if dystonia is the sole feature, and the anatomy is not grossly distorted, then DBS should be offered. When spasticity and dystonia coexist, an ITB trial should be performed. For the rest of the cases, careful discussion on the leading symptoms should guide the treatment.

Conflict of Interest We declare that we have no conflict of interest.

References

1. Capelle H, Krauss J (2009) Functional stereotactic procedures for treatment of secondary dystonia. In: Lozano A, Gildenberg P, Tasker R (eds) Textbook of stereotactic and functional neurosurgery. Springer, Berlin, pp 1835–1856
2. Eltahawy H, Saint-Cyr J, Giladi N, Lang A, Lozano A (2004) Primary dystonia is more responsive than secondary dystonia to pallidal interventions: outcome after pallidotomy or pallidal deep brain stimulation. Neurosurgery 54:613–621
3. Geyer HL, Bressman SB (2007) Diagnosis of dystonia. In: Warner TT, Bressman SB (eds) Clinical diagnosis and management of dystonia. Informa healthcare, London, pp 1–14
4. Iacono RP, Kuniyoshi SM, Lonser RR, Maeda G, Inae AM, Ashwal S (1996) Simultaneous bilateral pallidoansotomy for idiopathic dystonia musculorum deformans. Pediatr Neurol 14:145–148

5. Krause M, Fogel W, Kloss M, Rasche D, Volkmann J (2004) Pallidal stimulation for dystonia. Neurosurgery 55:1361–1370
6. Iacono RP, Kuniyoshi SM, Schoonenberg T (1998) Experience with stereotactics for dystonia: case examples. Adv Neurol 78: 221–226
7. Lin JJ, Lin SZ, Lin GY, Chang DC, Lee CC (1998) Application of bilateral sequential pallidotomy to treat a patient with generalized dystonia. Eur Neurol 40:108–110
8. Lin JJ, Lin GY, Shih C, Lin SZ, Chang DC, Lee CC (1999) Benefit of bilateral pallidotomy in the treatment of generalized dystonia: case report. J Neurosurg 90:974–976
9. Lozano AM, Kumar R, Gross RE, Giladi N, Hutchison WD, Dostrovsky JO, Lang AE (1997) Globus pallidus internus pallidotomy for generalized dystonia. Mov Disord 12:865–870
10. Vitek JL (1998) Surgery for dystonia. Neurosurg Clin N Am 9: 345–366
11. Vitek JL, Zhang J, Evatt M, Mewes K, DeLong MR, Hashimoto T, Triche S, Bakay RAE (1998) GPi pallidotomy for dystonia: clinical outcome and neuronal activity. Adv Neurol 78:211–219
12. Krauss JK, Yianni J, Loher TJ, Aziz TZ (2004) Deep brain stimulation for dystonia. J Clin Neurophysiol 21:18–30
13. Welter M, Grabli D, Vidailhet M (2010) Deep brain stimulation for hyperkinetic disorders: dystonia, tardive dyskinesia and tics. Curr Opin Neurol 23:420–425
14. Vercueil L, Pollak P, Fraix V, Caputo E, Moro E, Benazzouz A et al (2001) Deep brain stimulation in the treatment of severe dystonia. J Neurol 248:695–700
15. Cif L, El Fertit H, Vayssiere N, Hemm S, Hardouin E, Gannau A, Tuffery S, Coubes P (2003) Treatment of dystonic syndromes by chronic electrical stimulation of the internal globus pallidus. J Neurosurg Sci 47:52–55
16. Aziz T, Green A (2009) Dystonia: a surgeon's perspective. Parkinsonism Relat Disord 15S(3):S75–S80
17. Katsakiori PF, Kefalopoulou Z, Markaki E, Paschali A, Ellul J, Kagadis GC et al (2009) Deep brain stimulation for secondary dystonia: results in 8 patients. Acta Neurochir 151(5):473–478
18. Lin JJ, Lin SZ, Chang DC (1999) Pallidotomy and generalized dystonia. Mov Disord 14:1057–1059
19. Ondo WG, Krauss JK (2003) Surgical therapies for dystonia. In: Brin MF, Comella C, Jankovic J (eds) Dystonia monograph. Lippincott, Williams & Wilkins, Philadelphia, pp 125–147
20. Trottenberg T, Volkmann J, Deuschl G, Kuhn AA, Schneider GH, Muller J et al (2005) Treatment of severe tardive dystonia with pallidal deep brain stimulation. Neurology 64:344–346
21. Arnone D, Hansen L, Kerr JS (2002) Acute dystonic reaction in an elderly patient with mood disorder after titration of paroxetine: possible mechanisms and implications for clinical care. J Psychopharmacol 16:395–397
22. Sako W, Goto S, Shimazu H, Murase N, Matsuzaki K, Tamura T et al (2008) Bilateral deep brain stimulation of the globus pallidus internus in tardive dystonia. Mov Disord 23:1929–1931
23. Damier P, Thobois S, Witjas T, Cuny E, Derost P, Raoul S et al (2007) French Stimulation for Tardive Dyskinesia (STARDYS) Study Group. Bilateral deep brain stimulation of the globus pallidus to treat tardive dyskinesia. Arch Gen Psychiatry 64:170–176
24. Vidailhet M, Lagrannge C, Welter ML, Krack P, Krystowiak P, Burbaud P et al (2008) Bilateral pallidal stimulation in generalized dystonia related to post-anoxic birth injury: multicentre study. Mov Disord Suppl 1:162
25. Vidailhet M, Yelnik J, Lagrange C et al (2009) Bilateral pallidal deep brain stimulation for the treatment of patients with dystonia-choreoathetosis cerebral palsy: a prospective pilot study. Lancet Neurol 8:709–717
26. Krauss JK, Loher TJ, Weigel R, Capelle HH, Weber S, Burgunder JM (2003) Chronic stimulation of the globus pallidus internus for treatment of non-DYT1 generalized dystonia and choreoathetosis: 2-year follow up. J Neurosurg 98:785–792
27. Loher TJ, Hasdemir MG, Burgunder JM, Krauss JK (2000) Long-term follow-up study of chronic globus pallidus internus stimulation for posttraumatic hemidystonia. J Neurosurg 92:457–460
28. Yianni J, Bain P, Giladi N, Auca M, Gregory R, Joint C, Nandi D, Stein J, Scott R, Aziz T (2003) Globus pallidus internus deep brain stimulation for dystonic conditions: a prospective audit. Mov Disord 18:436–442
29. Motta F, Antonello C, Stignani C (2009) Upper limbs function after intrathecal baclofen therapy in children with secondary dystonia. J Pediatr Orthop 29:817–821
30. Butler C, Campbell S (2000) Evidence of the effects of intrathecal baclofen for spastic and dystonic cerebral palsy. Dev Med Child Neurol 42(9):634–645
31. Albright AL, Ferson SS (2006) Intrathecal baclofen therapy in children. Neurosurg Focus 21(2):e3
32. Narayan RK, Loubser PG, Jankovic J et al (1991) Intrathecal baclofen for intractable axial dystonia. Neurology 41(7):1141–1142
33. Penn RD, Gianino JM, York MM (1995) Intrathecal baclofen for motor disorders. Mov Disord 10(5):675–677
34. Ford B, Green P, Louis E, Petzinger G, Bressman S, Goodman R et al (1996) Use of intrathecal baclofen in the treatment of patients with dystonia. Arch Neurol 53:1241–1246
35. Albright AL, Barry MJ, Shafron DH, Ferson SS (2001) Intrathecal baclofen for generalized dystonia. Dev Med Child Neurol 43:652–657
36. Albright AL (1996) Intrathecal baclofen in cerebral palsy movement disorders. J Child Neurol 11:S29–S35
37. Albright AL, Barry MJ, Painter MJ, Shultz B (1998) Infusion of intrathecal baclofen for generalized dystonia in cerebral palsy. J Neurosurg 88:73–76
38. Motta F, Stignani C, Antonello CE (2008) Effect of intrathecal baclofen on dystonia in children with cerebral palsy and the use of functional scales. J Pediatr Orthop 28:213–217
39. Ward A, Hayden S, Dexter M, Scheinberg A (2009) Continuous intrathecal baclofen for children with spasticity and/or dystonia: goal attainment and complications associated with treatment. J Paediatr Child Health 45:720–726
40. Albright AL, Barry MJ, Fasick P, Barron W, Shultz B (1996) Continuous intrathecal baclofen infusion for symptomatic generalized dystonia. Neurosurgery 38:934–939
41. Albright AL (2007) Intrathecal baclofen for childhood hypertonia. Childs Nerv Syst 23:971–979
42. Albright AL (1996) Baclofen in the treatment of cerebral palsy. J Child Neurol 11(2):77–83

Deep Brain Stimulation of the Ventrolateral Thalamic Base and Posterior Subthalamic Area in Dystonic Head Tremor

Carsten Buhmann, Christian K.E. Moll, Simone Zittel, Alexander Münchau, Andreas K. Engel, and Wolfgang Hamel

Abstract Dystonic head tremor (DHT) is characterized by head tremor associated with cervical dystonia (CD). Deep brain stimulation (DBS) can be considered when local treatment with botulinum toxin or oral medication has failed. However, there is lack of data regarding the optimal target structure for surgery in DHT.

DBS of the ventrolateral (VL) thalamus is an established treatment option for medically refractory tremor. Tremor suppression is described as being most effective when stimulating at the inferior thalamic base and within the posterior subthalamic area (PSA). Moreover, there is surgical evidence from the pre-DBS era that both lesions and high-frequency stimulation of the PSA improve CD. Based on these observations, we performed DBS in three patients with DHT, placing the proximal contacts of the electrodes into the inferior base of VL thalamic nuclei and the distal contacts into the adjacent PSA. Chronic stimulation improved not only head tremor but also CD. These findings suggest that DBS at the base of VL thalamus and the adjacent PSA should undergo further investigation as a potential target for patients with DHT.

Keywords Cervical dystonia • Dystonic tremor • Head tremor • Deep brain stimulation

C. Buhmann, MD (✉), S. Zittel, MD, A. Münchau, MD, and W. Hamel, MD
Department of Neurology, University Medical Center Hamburg-Eppendorf, Martinistrasse 52, 20246 Hamburg, Germany
e-mail: buhmann@uke.uni-hamburg.de

C.K.E. Moll, MD and A.K. Engel, MD, PhD
Department of Neurophysiology and Pathophysiology, Center of Experimental Medicine, University Medical Center Hamburg-Eppendorf, Martinistrasse 52, 20246 Hamburg, Germany

Introduction

Dystonic head tremor (DHT) describes head tremor in patients with primary cervical dystonia (CD) [3, 4, 25]. DHT is found in 68 % of CD patients [22], and is less responsive to oral pharmacotherapy than hand tremor [6]. Local injections of botulinum toxin often improve not only CD but also tremor, but in some cases deep brain stimulation (DBS) might be considered. It is suggested that treatment of dystonic tremor matches the treatment of dystonia [6, 24], i.e., pallidal stimulation, although results in patients with DHT are conflicting and limited to case reports. We [18] and others [28] have reported on successful stimulation of the globus pallidus, pars interna (GPi) in single patients with DHT. In contrast, DHT was refractory to GPi stimulation in two other cases [16, 19].

We report on three patients with medically refractory DHT who underwent stereotactic implantation of quadropolar DBS electrodes. We aimed to place the upper contacts of the DBS lead at the base of the ventrolateral (VL) thalamus, and the lower contacts within the adjacent posterior subthalamic area (PSA). Our decision was driven by reports on excellent tremor suppression of different etiology by DBS at the VL thalamic base and within the PSA [8, 10], and relief of cervical dystonia by lesioning [17, 20, 21] and early explorative DBS [20] within the PSA.

Case histories, stereotactic localization of the most effective contacts, and clinical outcome are described, and results are discussed.

Patients and Methods

Patients

CD was rated according to the Toronto Western Spasmodic Torticollis Rating Scale, Part I — Torticollis Severity Scale (TWSTRS (I), maximal 35 points). Head tremor was evaluated

G. Nikkhah and M. Pinsker (eds.), *Stereotactic and Functional Neurosurgery*, Acta Neurochirurgica Supplement, Vol. 117,
DOI 10.1007/978-3-7091-1482-7_11, © Springer-Verlag Wien 2013

on the basis of the Fahn–Tolosa–Marin Tremor Rating scale, Part A, subitem 4: head tremor at rest (lying down), posture (when sitting or standing) and action (when turning); severity rating: 0 = none, 1 = slight; barely perceivable, 2 = moderate, may be intermittent, 3 = marked, 4 = severe (TRS (A) head, maximal 12 points). Clinical data of individual patients are summarized in Table 1.

Surgical Procedure

All patients described here underwent stereotactic bilateral implantation of DBS electrodes into the inferior base of VL thalamus and adjacent PSA. Operative interventions were performed in local anaesthesia as described previously [7, 18]. The surgical target was defined 6–7 mm posterior and 12.5–13.5 mm lateral to the midcommissural point. Surgery included simultaneous microrecordings from 2 to 3 microelectrodes (MicroGuide, Alpha–Omega, Nazareth, Israel) in steps of 250–500 μm using a Ben's gun approach to map kinetic and tremor-related cells and the inferior border of the thalamus. Macrostimulation via the uninsulated distal end of the guide tube was performed intraoperatively to identify the trajectory resulting in most effective tremor suppression which was associated with the least adverse effects. We intended to position at least two contacts of the quadropolar 3389 electrodes (Medtronic Inc. Minneapolis, MN, USA) within the PSA. At the end of the operative procedure, both DBS electrodes were test-stimulated to assess side-effects. Tremor had subsided in most cases due to a microlesioning effect and could not be assessed further. Stimulator implantation (model Kinetra or PC, Medtronic Inc.) was performed in general anaesthesia on the same day or on the day following electrode implantation.

We employed intraoperative computerized tomography scanning (CT, Siemens Somatom with sliding-gantry system, Erlangen, Germany) to determine the position of the implanted electrodes. Stereotactic CT images (1 mm slice thickness; window center 80 HU, 'width' 95–100 HU; matrix 512 × 512 pixel; FOV 280 mm) covering the distal >30 mm of the implanted electrodes were obtained while the stereotactic frame (Zamorano-Dujovny; Stryker-Leibinger, Freiburg, Germany) was left in place. The postoperative CT scans were co-registered with preoperative CT and magnetic resonance images (MRI).

Results

All patients had inconspicuous family history for tremor and dystonia. Tremor was in part relieved by alcohol in cases 1 and 3. Preoperatively, treatment with oral medication and electromyography (EMG)-guided local botulinum toxin injections up to occurrence of side-effects was largely ineffective. MRI was inconspicuous in all patients.

Following bilateral electrode implantation into the base of VL thalamus and adjacent PSA, chronic stimulation improved tremor and cervical dystonia in all cases. Coordinates of clinically effective electrode contacts and programming parameters are provided in Table 2. The following section contains the detailed case presentations.

Case 1

This 39-year-old male patient presented with a 26-year history of initial arm tremor followed by head twisting and trembling. On examination, he had DHT (CD with torti- and laterocollis to the left) with a positive geste antagonistique associated with an irregular, kinetic head tremor (mainly 'yes–yes' direction) and a position-specific severe jerky component when leaning the head backwards. Furthermore, he had mild dysarthria and a slight and not disabling action tremor of both hands (TWSTRS (I) 8 points, TRS (A) head 6 points; Table 1). Surface EMG of right sternocleidomastoid and upper trapezius muscles showed a mixture of regular and irregular bursts with a duration of 100 ms or longer. Epsilon sarcoglycan gene mutation was negative. Postoperatively dysarthria and CD were unchanged. Microlesioning resulted in a complete cessation of the tremulous head motion, which lasted up to 16 days. Consequently, the head tremor progressively re-appeared. Monopolar stimulation performed bilaterally with the second most distal contacts (i.e., contacts 1- and 9- cathodal vs case + anode) improved symptoms markedly (TWSTRS (I) 1 points, TRS (A) head 2 points), but induced a slight increase of dysarthria and imbalance. Therefore, 3 months postoperatively the active contacts were changed bilaterally to the second most proximal contacts (contacts 2- and 10-; Table 2). Stimulation in the left hemisphere was continued in the PSA; however, stimulation on the right side was at the base of the thalamus (Table 2). This resulted in lasting improvement of DHT without side-effects for more than 20 months. Whereas tremor immediately improved after the initiation of stimulation, CD improved progressively over a time period of 3–5 months.

Case 2

This 66-year-old female patient presented with a 10-year history of head trembling and involuntary turning of the head to the right. On examination, she had mild and intermittent right torticollis and a slight lateral shift to the left associated with an irregular and position specific 4–5 Hz DHT (predominantly 'yes–yes' direction). Both abnormal head posture and DHT were improved by touching the chin with one finger. Holding the arms straight forward, a slight dystonic finger posture on the left was present (TWSTRS (I) 7 points, TRS (A) head 5 points).

In contrast to the other patients, postoperatively no relevant microlesioning effect could be observed. Permanent monopolar stimulation of contacts '2' and '9' was performed

Table 1 Provides patient details

Pat.	Sex	Age at surgery (years)	Disease duration at surgery (years)	Affected body parts	Alcohol response of tremor	Medication pre-OP (dose/day) (MU BTX)	Medication post-OP (dose/day) (MU BTX)	TWSTRS (I) pre-OP	TWSTRS (I) post-OP	TRS (A) head pre-OP	TRS (A) head post-OP	Postoperative follow-up (months)
1	M	39	26	Cervical and slightly both upper extremities	Yes	Propranolol 240 mg Primidone 250 mg Gabapentine 900 mg Trihexiphenidyl 14 mg Clonazepam 6 mg Topiramat 100 mg Antidepressiva, NA Botox® 100MU, 2× Xeomin® 120MU, 2×	None	8	1	6	2	20
2	F	66	10	Cervical	No	Propranolol 120 mg Primidone 250 mg Gabapentine 900 mg Biperidin 15 mg Lamotrigine 100 mg Botox® 120MU, 2×	None	7	2	5	2	18
3	M	54	16	Cervical and slightly both upper extremities	Yes	Metoprolol 95 mg Primidone 250 mg Clozapin 25 mg Topiramat 100 mg Dysport® up to 640MU, 5× Botox® 65MU, 1× Neurobloc® 8400MU, 1×	None	10	4	8	3	13

Pre- and postoperative medication and TWSTRS (I) and TRS (A) head score (subitem 4) are listed at the thalamic base on both sides (Table 2). Stimulation through the more distal contacts also resulted in efficient tremor suppression, but induced disturbing dysarthria. Tremor improved within a few days after initiation of stimulation, CD within the first 3 months. Best results were seen with stimulation at the VL thalamic base on both sides (Table 2). Clinical improvement was stable, and was rated after18 months (TWSTRS (I) 2 points, TRS head (A) 2 points; Table 1).

Case 3

This 54-year-old male patient presented with head tremor started 16 years ago, followed by involuntary head turning 2–3 years later. Slight bilateral postural hand tremor appeared 2 years prior to surgery. On examination, he had mild torticollis to the left (30°) and mild laterocollis to the right (15°) and moderate to severe slightly irregular and position specific DHT of high frequency (6–8 Hz) but low amplitude (exclusively 'no–no' direction). Geste antagonistique was positive for both abnormal head posture and DHT. Additionally, a postural arm tremor of rather high frequency and low amplitude without intention tremor was present (TWSTRS (I) 10 points, TRS head (A) 8 points). Permanent monopolar stimulation of the second most distal contacts '1' and '9', located in the PSA, proved to be most effective and without adverse effects (Table 2). CD and DHT showed stable improvement as documented 13 months postoperatively (TWSTRS (I) 4 points, TRS (A) head 3; Table 2).

Discussion

Classification of head tremor associated with CD is not unambiguous [3, 25]. The patients reported here all presented with both CD and associated head tremor, and their condition was classified as dystonic head tremor [3, 4, 25]. Diagnosis of DHT is supported by reduction of head tremor amplitude during a geste antagonistique maneuver [5, 12] and presence of a neck position-specific tremor component or a jerky, irregular tremor [3, 13] with rhythmic expression of rapid dystonic movements. As observed in two of our patients, tremor relief through alcohol can not only be seen in essential tremor but also in DHT [12].

Selection of the DBS target in DHT is mainly driven by individual characteristics of the dystonic tremor rather than based on clear-cut clinical disease classification. Furthermore, there is lack of clinical studies comparing the efficacy of potential targets for DHT, i.e., VL thalamus, PSA and GPi. We decided to place the electrodes with the lower contacts within the PSA and the upper contacts at the base of VL thalamus as delineated by intraoperative microelectrode recordings. In all our three DHT patients, bilateral DBS did not only improve tremor but also CD. Stereotactic localization demonstrated an even distribution of clinically effective electrode contacts between VL thalamus and PSA (Table 2). The stereotactic coordinates of the electrodes implanted are presented in Table 2.

Two recent case series documented successful thalamic DBS in two [27] and three [19] patients with severe dystonic tremor, two of them with DHT [19]. In addition, stimulation of structures within the PSA have been reported to improve various dystonic tremor syndromes [1, 14, 23], including one case with symptomatic DHT after perinatal anoxia [14]. In one case, bilateral DBS of the subthalamic nucleus has been reported to completely suppress tremor and nearly resolve CD in a patient with DHT and action tremor of the hands [2]. However, the localization of the active electrode contacts was not reported.

The PSA is an anisotropic region in which different systems intersect. Whereas cerebellothalamic projections within the PSA may represent the relevant substrate for the surgical relief of tremor, modulation of pallidofugal fibres within the PSA may bring out the beneficial effects on dystonic symptoms. Pallidofugal fibres of the ansa lenticularis and the lenticular fasciculus (Forel's field H2) join in Forel's field H before entering the thalamus in Forel's field H1 [15, 26]. Within the PSA, the zona incerta (ZI) conveys afferents from the interstitial nucleus of Cajal. It has been known for a long time that stimulation of this nucleus as well as stimulation within the ZI may induce head rotation in animals [9, 11]. Moreover the ZI receives afferents from GPi and substantia nigra, pars reticulata and sends efferents to the ventroanterior and VL thalamic nuclei (overview in [23]).

Taken together, the intricate anatomical relationships at the thalamic base with its high density of different fiber systems and interconnected nuclei put any operative intervention in the thalamic base/PSA border zone in the position of "bottle-neck surgery". Along with this, we found the most effective and therefore active electrodes for tremor and dystonia relief to be located in the VL thalamic base ($n=3$) as well as in the adjacent PSA ($n=3$). So the "bottle-neck" approach may help to explain the efficacy of the PSA as surgical target in a variety of disease entities, such as different tremors, Parkinson's disease and dystonia.

General conclusions from this case series are limited due to the small sample size. Hitherto, reports on DBS in patients with DHT have been rare. Patients reported here expressed relatively more tremor than dystonia. Therefore effects of DBS in the VL thalamic base/PSA in DHT patients with more severe dystonic symptoms remain to be evaluated. A prospective and controlled study with separate investigations of all contacts on tremor and dystonia in a blinded fashion is desirable.

Table 2 Describes individual anatomical and microrecording parameters as well as localization and stimulation parameters of the active electrodes

Pat.	Location of active electrode	Stimulation parameters (hemisphere)	Width of 3 ventricle (mm)	Length AC-PC (mm)	*Z* level of VL thalamic base according to microelectrodes recording	*x*/*y*/*z* coordinates of active electrodes in mm (hemisphere)
1	PSA	Left: 2–/C+, 1.5 V, 60 µs, 180 Hz	2.0	25.1	n/a	Left: −9.3/−5.8/−2.6
	VL thalamic base	Right: 10–/C+, 1,5 V, 60 µs, 180 Hz			−0.7	Right: +10.7/−3.7/+0.7
2	VL thalamic base	Left: 2–/C+, 2,4 V, 90 µs, 160 Hz	11.0	24.8	−0.3	Left: −12.3/−6.2/−0.9
	VL thalamic base	Right: 9–/C+, 2,2 V, 90 µs, 160 Hz			−0.4	Right: +13.4/−6.2/+0.6
3	PSA	Left: 1–/C+, 2,0 V, 60 µs, 130 Hz	4.0	23.1	−0.6	Left: −8.9/−4.6/−4.7
	PSA	Right 9–/C+, 2,0 V, 60 µs, 130 Hz			0.8	Right: +8.3/−6.5/−3.0

x/*y*/*z* coordinates (center of single electrode contact — Medtronic 3389; length: 1.5 mm) and *z*-level in relation to the midcommissural point (MCP)
PSA posterior subthalamic area, *VL* ventrolateral, *MCP* Midpoint of the anterior–posterior commissural line (AC-PC), *C* case, '–' cathodal, '+' anodal

Financial Disclosure and Potential Conflict of Interest The authors have occasionally received travel expenses and honoraria from Medtronic Inc. for speaking at meetings.

References

1. Blomstedt P, Sandvik U, Tisch S (2010) Deep brain stimulation in the posterior subthalamic area in the treatment of essential tremor. Mov Disord 25(10):1350–1356
2. Chou KL, Hurtig HI, Jaggi JL, Baltuch GH (2005) Bilateral subthalamic nucleus deep brain stimulation in a patient with cervical dystonia and essential tremor. Mov Disord 20(3):377–380
3. Deuschl G (2003) Dystonic tremor. Rev Neurol (Paris) 159(10 Pt 1): 900–905
4. Deuschl G, Bain P, Brin M (1998) Consensus statement of the Movement Disorder Society on Tremor. Ad Hoc Scientific Committee. Mov Disord 13(Suppl 3):2–23
5. Deuschl G, Heinen F, Kleedorfer B, Wagner M, Lucking CH, Poewe W (1992) Clinical and polymyographic investigation of spasmodic torticollis. J Neurol 239(1):9–15
6. Gironell A, Kulisevsky J (2009) Diagnosis and management of essential tremor and dystonic tremor. Ther Adv Neurol Disord 2(4):215–222
7. Hamel W, Fietzek U, Morsnowski A, Schrader B, Herzog J, Weinert D, Pfister G, Muller D, Volkmann J, Deuschl G, Mehdorn HM (2003) Deep brain stimulation of the subthalamic nucleus in Parkinson's disease: evaluation of active electrode contacts. J Neurol Neurosurg Psychiatry 74(8):1036–1046
8. Hamel W, Herzog J, Kopper F, Pinsker M, Weinert D, Muller D, Krack P, Deuschl G, Mehdorn HM (2007) Deep brain stimulation in the subthalamic area is more effective than nucleus ventralis intermedius stimulation for bilateral intention tremor. Acta Neurochir (Wien) 149(8):749–758
9. Hassler R (1954) Experimentelle und anatomische Befunde über die Drehbewegungen und ihre nervösen Apparate. Arch Psychiat Nervenkr 192:488–526
10. Hassler R (1965) Correlations between clinical and autoptic findings in stereotaxic operations of parkinsonism. Confin Neurol 26:282–290
11. Hyde JE, Toczek S (1962) Functional relation of interstitial nucleus to rotatory movements evoked from zona incerta stimulation. J Neurophysiol 25:455–466
12. Jankovic J, Leder S, Warner D, Schwartz K (1991) Cervical dystonia: clinical findings and associated movement disorders. Neurology 41(7):1088–1091
13. Jedynak CP, Bonnet AM, Agid Y (1991) Tremor and idiopathic dystonia. Mov Disord 6(3):230–236
14. Jeong SG, Lee MK, Lee WH, Ghang CG (2009) Deep brain stimulation of the subthalamic area for dystonic tremor. J Korean Neurosurg Soc 45(5):303–305
15. Jones EG (1985) The thalamus. Plenum Press, New York
16. Krause M, Fogel W, Kloss M, Rasche D, Volkmann J, Tronnier V (2004) Pallidal stimulation for dystonia. Neurosurgery 55(6): 1361–1368
17. Moll CK, Hamel W, Ostertag CB, Muller D, Finsterbusch J, Engel AK, Munchau A (2008) Subthalamotomy in cervical dystonia: a case study of lesion location and clinical outcome. Mov Disord 23(12):1751–1756
18. Moll CK, Sharott A, Hamel W, Munchau A, Buhmann C, Hidding U, Zittel S, Westphal M, Muller D, Engel AK (2009) Waking up the brain: a case study of stimulation-induced wakeful unawareness during anaesthesia. Prog Brain Res 177:125–145
19. Morishita T, Foote KD, Haq IU, Zeilman P, Jacobson CE, Okun MS (2010) Should we consider Vim thalamic deep brain stimulation for select cases of severe refractory dystonic tremor. Stereotact Funct Neurosurg 88(2):98–104
20. Mundinger F (1977) New stereotactic treatment of spasmodic torticollis with a brain stimulation system (author's transl). Med Klin 72(46):1982–1986
21. Mundinger F, Riechert T, Disselhoff J (1972) Long-term results of stereotactic treatment of spasmodic torticollis. Confin Neurol 34(2): 41–50
22. Pal PK, Samii A, Schulzer M, Mak E, Tsui JK (2000) Head tremor in cervical dystonia. Can J Neurol Sci 27(2):137–142
23. Plaha P, Khan S, Gill SS (2008) Bilateral stimulation of the caudal zona incerta nucleus for tremor control. J Neurol Neurosurg Psychiatry 79(5):504–513
24. Raethjen J (2011) Current therapy for tremor. Aktuelle Neurol 38(6): 315–319
25. Rivest J, Marsden CD (1990) Trunk and head tremor as isolated manifestations of dystonia. Mov Disord 5(1):60–65
26. von Monakow C (1895) Experimentelle und pathologisch-anatomische Untersuchungen über die Haubenregion, den Sehhügel und die Regio subthalamica, nebst Beiträgen zur Kenntnis früh erworbener Gross und Kleinhirndefecte. Arch Psychiatr Nervenkr 27:1–128, 386–478
27. Woehrle JC, Blahak C, Kekelia K, Capelle HH, Baezner H, Grips E, Weigel R, Krauss JK (2009) Chronic deep brain stimulation for segmental dystonia. Stereotact Funct Neurosurg 87(6):379–384
28. Yianni J, Nandi D, Hyam J, Elliott V, Bain P, Gregory R, Aziz T (2004) Failure of chronic pallidal stimulation in dystonic patients is a medical emergency. Neuromodulation 7(1):9–12

Intra-operative Transdural Electric Stimulation in Awake Patient: Target Refining for Motor Cortex Stimulation

Manoel Jacobsen Teixeira, Daniel Ciampi de Andrade, and Erich Talamoni Fonoff

Abstract *Introduction.* Most authors perform the implantation of epidural electrodes for motor cortex stimulation (MCS) under general anesthesia, using navigation merely based on anatomic landmarks or in combination with intra-operative sensory evoked potentials (SEP) for functional localization. However, intra-operative SEP can only provide the localization of central sulcus in patients who present sensory pathways which are at least partially preserved. Conversely, there are massive deafferentation pain syndromes (e.g., brachial plexus avulsion or amputation) in which the peripheral sensory pathways are severely or totally injured, precluding the use of intra-operative SEP.

Objective. The authors present a simple technique for functional localization and intra-operative mapping of motor cortex by the implementation of transdural electrical stimulation of cerebral cortex for target refining of motor cortex during cortical electrode implantation procedures.

Methods. Thirteen patients with complete brachial plexus root avulsion suffering from severe neuropathic pain in the affected limb were included in this report. First, the anatomical location of the motor cortex of the hand was stereotactically determined by the hand knob within the central sulcus. Functional mapping of cortex was performed by transdural bipolar electrical stimulation under local anesthesia, so patients were fully awake during the whole time of cortical mapping. The cortical mapping oriented the placement of epidural electrodes for chronic cortical stimulation for treatment of neuropathic pain.

Results. Stereotactic MR images of the hand knob were considered a satisfactory landmark for the motor area of the hand in all patients. On top of the anatomical landmark, transdural electrical stimulation (4.0–6.0 mA, 30–60 Hz and pulse width of 1 ms) gave vivid sensations of movement in the deafferented hand, forearm, and arm. The phantom sensation was elicited with lower current than usual motor mapping in patients with intact limbs. It was possible to delineate the spatial map of the phantom hand on the cortical surface with acceptable resolution. The sensation of wrist flexion was elicited in all; most of the patients had clear distinction of the thumb and index. The remaining fingers were not perceived individually. The cortical area responsive to the thumb tended to occupy a lateral position related to the areas of the other fingers, following the maps of the normal homunculus. The evoked sensation was restricted to the period of stimulation, and it stopped as soon as that was discontinued. The stimulation also evoked emotional responses related to sensation of limb movement.

Conclusion. The proposed technique was useful for target refining in implantation of epidural electrode for motor cortex stimulation. Further studies are required to investigate if target refining by intra-operative mapping will significantly improve the results in the treatment of refractory pain.

Keywords Motor cortex stimulation • Cortical mapping • Pain • Cerebral cortex • Intraoperative neurophysiology

Introduction

Since the first reports, motor cortex stimulation (MCS) has gained much enthusiasm in the literature as a treatment for refractory neuropathic pain [17]. Although the efficacy of MCS has been questioned because of variable results, hundreds of patients around the world have been benefited by this technique in the treatment of refractory pain. Good results have been achieved in various pain syndromes: trigeminal neuralgia, trigeminal neuropathy [10–12] phantom limb pain

M.J. Teixeira, MD, PhD, D.C. de Andrade, MD, PhD, and E.T. Fonoff, MD, PhD (✉)
Pain Center and Division of Functional Neurosurgery, Department of Neurology, School of Medicine of University of São Paulo, Rua Dr. Ovídio Pires de Campos, 785, São Paulo, SP 01060-970, Brazil
e-mail: fonoffet@usp.br

G. Nikkhah and M. Pinsker (eds.), *Stereotactic and Functional Neurosurgery*, Acta Neurochirurgica Supplement, Vol. 117,
DOI 10.1007/978-3-7091-1482-7_12, © Springer-Verlag Wien 2013

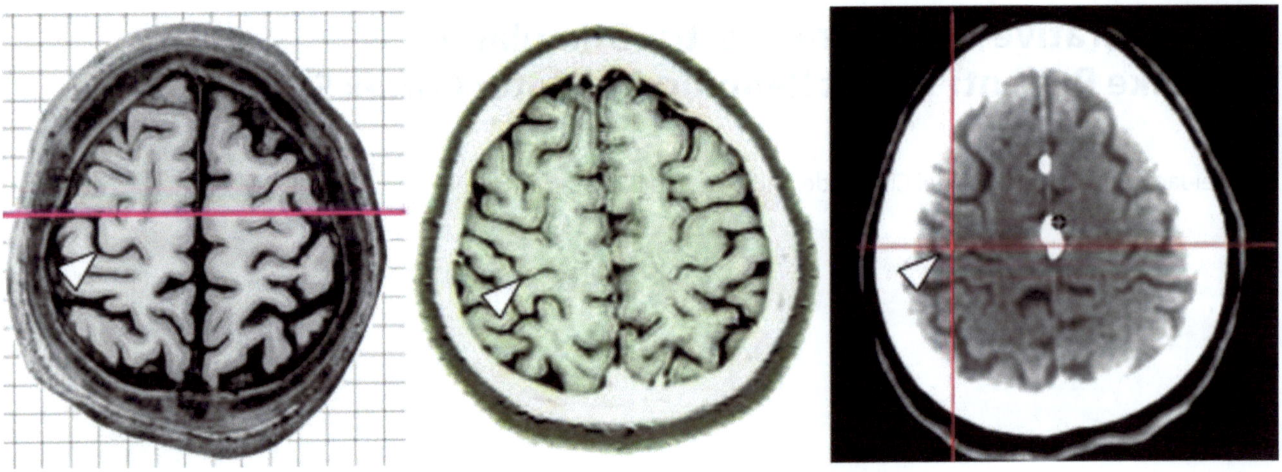

Fig. 1 Illustration of the omega shaped knob of precentral gyrus (*white arrowhead*) with central sulcus, referred to as the hand knob, or the primary motor area of the hand in horizontal section of anatomical slices (*left*), magnetic resonance image (*center*) and computed tomography (*right*). The figures illustrate that the hand knob may vary in shape from *omega* to *epsilon*

[16] post stroke pain [18], and complex regional pain syndrome [6, 19] among other deafferentation pain syndromes.

However, the best approach to determine the site for implanting MCS electrodes is still a matter of debate. Most of the authors perform the implantation procedure under general anesthesia, using different methods for the localization of motor cortex. Reports include either localization of precentral gyrus based merely on anatomic landmarks, or added to intra-operative sensory evoked potentials (SEP) for functional localization. Intra-operative SEP is oriented for the localization of central sulcus and consequently the precentral gyrus. The combination of those techniques provides the functional localization of the precentral gyrus corresponding to the motor cortex, limited to patients who present sensory pathways which are at least partially preserved. On the other hand, there are deafferentation pain syndromes (e.g., brachial plexus avulsion or amputation) in which the peripheral sensory pathways are severely or totally injured, precluding the intra-operative use of SEP for target refining.

The authors present a simple technique that can provide detailed functional and spatial information for target refining in implantation of motor cortex stimulation electrodes for the treatment of pain. The procedure performed in an awake patient provides the possibility of mapping the motor cortex in either amputees or injured plexus patients, evoking phantom sensation by transdural electrical stimulation of the cerebral cortex.

Methods

Thirteen patients with severe neuropathic pain in upper limb related to brachial plexus avulsion injury underwent implantation of MCS electrodes according to the technique proposed by the authors. The present technique relies on stereotactic localization of the hand knob in the posterior aspects of the precentral gyrus based in the MRI to guide the starting point for intra-operative target refining by transdural stimulation of the cerebral cortex in awake patients.

Surgical Procedure and Intra-operative Localization of the Motor Cortex

Standard framed stereotactic computed tomography (CT) images fused to the MR images in a dedicated computer graphic software (MICROMAR Stereotactic Assistant — MSA) were used to guide the localization of the central sulcus and the precentral gyrus. The center of the omega-shaped knob on the posterior border of the pre-central gyrus within the central sulcus, lining with the superior frontal sulcus, was the intended anatomic landmark used to guide the initial point in the surface of *dura* for electrical stimulation mapping. As suggested by Yousry et al. [22], the image generated by this knob in the horizontal MR images is highly specific to indicate the primary motor area of hand in normal subjects. However, this point is usually 1.5–2 cm deep into the central sulcus and 3.5 cm from midline. The coordinates of the hand knob were then projected onto the surface of the scalp to guide the skin incision, further projected onto the surface of the skull to point the center of the craniotomy, and finally the same projection was made onto the dural surface in order to provide the initial point for cortical mapping by transdural electrical stimulation. A small craniotomy (3 cm) encompassing the region of the anatomical target was then carried out under local anesthesia and light sedation (Fig. 1).

After the craniotomy was performed, sedation was then completely withdrawn so the patient was completely awake.

The patient's awakefulness was tested by simple temporo-spatial orientation questions. Transdural bipolar stimulation of the cortex was conducted at amplitudes up to 4–6 mA, 1 ms and 30–60 Hz (Micromar AC Cortical Stimulator, São Paulo, Brazil). As the stimulation session started, the patient was allowed to describe any sensation different from the resting status, after each short period of stimulation (1–2 s) in each site. The sites of stimulation were previous determined by a matrix of points that covered the surface of the exposed *dura*. Stimulation was then repeated in targets that generated any sensation of interest over a longer period (up to 5 s). The repeated stimulation allowed patients to improve the description of the sensation in a more detailed manner, including the part of the limb involved. To help the description of movements and the joints involved, as well as the speed and repetition of the entire movement, the patient used the contralateral limb to mimic the sensation of movement on the affected side.

Once mapping was finished, an epidural paddle electrode (Resume II, model 3587A, Medtronic, Minneapolis, MN, USA) was implanted following the map generated over the area of the greatest evoked motor sensation. The center contacts of the paddle electrode were placed over the area which elicited sensations topographically related to the area affected by the pain syndrome. The contacts in the two extremities of the electrode covered adjacent areas of the motor cortex also elicited by stimulation, the forearm, arm, face and so on.

Results

The CT-MRI image of the hand knob was a satisfactory anatomical parameter to find the motor area of the hand in all the patients. The electrical stimulation at 4.0–6.0 mA, 30–60 Hz, and 1 ms of pulse width evoked a vivid sensation of movement in the nonexistent hand, forearm, and arm. In these patients, the phantom movement exceeded the physical limits of existing and non-functional limb. The spatial map of the phantom hand on cortical surface could be delineated with good resolution. The sensation of wrist flexion was elicited in all patients; 61.3 % of the patients (8/13) had clear distinction of the thumb and index which was clearly different from the wrist flexion and from the other fingers. Phantom movements of the remaining fingers (third to fifth) were elicited in only 38.4 % of the patients (3/13). None of the patients referred a sensation of one finger in three separately, they were always sensed together. The cortical area responsive to thumb tended to occupy a lateral position related to the areas of the other fingers, following the maps of normal homunculus. The evoked sensation was restricted to the period of stimulation, and it stopped as soon as that was discontinued. The transdural stimulation map permitted the localization of the specific area of cortex related to the most severe pain. It was possible to cover this area also by the electrode contacts. The stimulation evoked emotional responses related to sensation of limb movement. We observed improvement of pain in nine of 13 patients (69.2 %). About 61.3 % had an over-50 % improvement of pain.

Discussion

The loss of peripheral feedback to the CNS and its related changes in cortical and subcortical organization of body representation have been reported to be the neurophysiologic basis of phantom limb phenomenon [5, 8]. Interestingly, not only amputees, but also conditions such as paraplegia or spinal anesthesia, brachial plexus root avulsion, or brachial plexus anesthetic block [7] may elicit phantom limb sensation as well as its motor component, phantom movements. These events range from eventual unwilling sensations to totally constant and voluntary phantom limb movements. At first glance, phantom movements seem to be phenomenologically related to imaginary movements of normal limbs. However, patients who experience both state that the sensation involved in each of the two is remarkably different. Investigation of phantom motor events is often difficult because of its highly subjective attributes. In order to minimize the subjectivity, Flor et al. proposed controlled and outpaced tasks during image data acquisition [5]. In such experiments, specific tasks are temporally correlated to the changes in brain metabolism (PET Scan), regional blood flow (SPECT), magnetic field potentials [21], or BOLD effect (fMRI). Recent works, mainly using fMRI and PET, have reported that voluntary phantom limb movement activates various cortical areas [4, 15]. However, Lotze et al. [9] have verified a larger activation on cortical areas during phantom motor phenomenon when compared to cortical activation in healthy subjects [2, 9]. This suggests that in some subjects, even if cortical reorganization takes place, cortical areas related to amputated limbs may be preserved or even enlarged, instead of fading out with time. Although the relationship to the presence of pain and the use of functional prosthetic devices has been reported, the mechanisms explaining this phenomenon are still undetermined [9].

Still relying on patient reports of subjective experiences, some investigators have approached this issue from another point of view. Either electrical or magnetic stimulation (TMS) may be applied to brain areas of fully awake patients producing tactile, auditive, or visual sensations, speech arrest, muscle contractions and even limb movements. This kind of procedure is routinely performed, for example, in functional neurosurgery for movement disorders or pain, cortical mapping for tumor resection [13] and epilepsy surgery [14], and also during TMS sessions [1]. Investigation of phantom limb phenomenon relies exactly on this kind of technique, because no electrophysiological recording can be performed on the amputed limb. Direct stimulation of thalamic nucleus has been found to elicit phantom sensitive phenomenon during intraoperative microelectrode recording and stimulation [3]. Ojeman et al. have performed direct stimulation of cortex during a ressective tumor surgery in an upper limb amputee. He found a well-defined sensory phenomenon when postcentral gyrus was stimulated, but no response during stimulation of precentral gyrus [13]. Woosley et al. also have performed direct cortical stimulation in two patients with phantom limb pain, reporting widening of the phantom limb corresponding area. The responses elicited were pain, sensitivity, and vague motor sensations on the amputated limb [20]. Amassian et al. described sensation of movement during magnetic coil stimulation of motor cortex in volunteers with blocked arm [1]. Cohen et al. reported that transcranial magnetic stimulation (TMS) may induce sensations of movement in the missing limb or fingers in patients with acquired amputation [2]. However, the motor sensation described by the subjects during single-shot magnetic stimulation were focal and ephemeral, generating poor descriptions [2] (Table 1).

In this report, the authors describe patient experiences during cortical mapping by transdural electric stimulation used to refine the target for implantation of motor cortex stimulation. The intraoperative cortical stimulation was used to refine the target for electrode implantation. This procedure was performed under local anesthesia in fully awake patients. This way, they could give a more detailed description of the phantom sensation including movement, comparing with motor imaginary on the normal side.

In conclusion, the proposed technique was useful for target refining of motor cortex stimulation. Further studies are required to investigate whether target refining by intra-operative mapping will significantly improve results in the treatment of refractory pain.

Table 1 Clinical and demographic data related to patient outcome and phantom limb phenomenon and elicited by intraoperative stimulation

Gender/age	Sensitive and motor root affected	Localization of pain	side	McGill description terms	Previous VAS	Previous procedures	Intraoperative mapping	Evoked phenomenon	Relief of pain (VAS) (%)	Phantom changes
M23	C5–T1	Hand and forearm	Left	Stabbing, burning, beating, throbbing	6	TENS, acup, anest blocks	Low threshold	Phantom movements	90	Increased vividness
M20	C5–T1	Cervical, arm and forearm	Right	Electric shock, stabbing	10	TENS, acup, anest blocks	High threshold	Small amplitude movements	Unchanged	No phantom
M27	C5–T1	Hand and forearm and arm	Right	Electric shock, crushing, burning	10	Anest blocks, neurolysis, SCS, micr. grafting, DREZotomy	High threshold	Phantom movements	Unchanged	No phantom
M47	C5–T1	Hand and forearm and arm	Right	Heavy stabbing, burning	10	TENS, acup, neurolysis, micr. grafting, SCS, DREZotomy	Low threshold	Small amplitude movements	75	Increased vividness
M39	C5–T1	Hand and forearm and arm	Left	Electric shock, crushing, burning	10	Neurolysis, micr. grafting, DREZotomy	Low threshold	Phantom movements	80	Vividness
M28	C5–T1	Hand and forearm	Left	Pulsing, electric shock, burning	10	TENS, acup, anest block, neurolysis micr. grafting, DREZotomy	Low threshold	Phantom movements	85	No changes
M29	C6–C8	Hand and forearm and arm	Right	Burning, electric shock, heavy	10	Anest blocks, neurolysis, SCS	Low threshold	Phantom movements	70	Increased vividness
M42	C5–T1	Hand and forearm and arm	Right	Burning, electric shock, heavy	10	Anest blocks, neurolysis, SCS	Low threshold	Phantom movements	60	
M52	C5–T1	Hand and forearm	Right	Stabbing, burning, throbbing	9	Drez	Phantom movs	Phantom movements	70	No changes
M46	C5–c8	Hand and forearm	Left	Burning	8	Acup, anest blocks	High threshold	Phantom movs	Unchanged	No changes
M50	C5–c8	Hand and forearm and arm	Left	Burning, electric shock	9	Drez	High threshold	Phantom limb	Unchanged	No changes
M32	C5–T1	Hand and forearm	Right	Burning, electric shock	10	Anest blocks, neurolysis	Low threshold	Phantom movs	70–80	
F36	C5–T1	Hand and forearm and arm	Right	Burning, electric shock	10	Anest block, neurolysis	Low threshold	Phantom movs	30	

Conflict of Interest The authors state that they have no conflict of interest related to this article.

References

1. Amassian VE, Cracco RQ, Maccabee PJ (1989) A sense of movement elicited in paralyzed distal arm by focal magnetic coil stimulation of human motor cortex. Brain Res 479:355–360
2. Cohen LG, Bandinelli S, Findley TW, Hallett M (1991) Motor reorganization after upper limb amputation in man. A study with focal magnetic stimulation. Brain 114:615–627
3. Davis KD, Kiss ZH, Luo L, Tasker RR, Lozano AM, Dostrovsky JO (1998) Phantom sensations generated by thalamic microstimulation. Nature 391:385–387
4. Dettmers C, Adler T, Rzanny R, Van Schayck R, Gaser C, Weiss T, Miltner WH, Bruckner L, Weiller C (2001) Increased excitability in the primary motor cortex and supplementary motor area in patients with phantom limb pain after upper limb amputation. Neurosci Lett 307:109–112
5. Flor H, Elbert T, Knecht S, Wienbruch C, Pantev C, Birbaumer N, Larbig W, Taub E (1995) Phantom-limb pain as a perceptual correlate of cortical reorganization following arm amputation. Nature 375:482–484
6. Fonoff ET, Hamani C, Andrade DC, Yeng LT, Marcolin MA, Teixeira MJ (2011) Pain relief and functional recovery in patients with complex regional pain syndrome after motor cortex stimulation. Stereotact Funct Neurosurg 89:167–172
7. Gentili ME, Verton C, Kinirons B, Bonnet F (2002) Clinical perception of phantom limb sensation in patients with brachial plexus blocks. Eur J Anaesthesiol 19:105–108
8. Lotze WM, Flor H, Grodd W, Larbig W, Birbaumer N (2001) Phantom movements and pain. An FMRI study in upper limb amputees. Brain 124:2268–2277
9. Lotze WM, Grodd N, Birbaumer M, Erb E, Huse E, Flor H (1999) Does use of a myoelectric prosthesis prevents cortical reorganization and phantom limb pain? Nat Neurosci 2(6):501–502
10. Meyerson BA, Lindblom U, Linderoth B, Lind G, Herregodts P (1993) Motor cortex stimulation as treatment of trigeminal neuropathic pain. Acta Neurochir Suppl (Wien) 58:150–153
11. Meyerson B (2005) Motor cortex stimulation-effective for neuropathic pain but the mode of action remains illusive. Pain 118:6–7
12. Nguyen JP, Lefaucheur JP, Decq P, Uchiyama T, Carpentier A, Fontaine D, Brugieres P, Pollin B, Feve A, Rostaing S, Cesaro P, Keravel Y (1999) Chronic motor cortex stimulation in the treatment of central and neuropathic pain. Correlations between clinical, electrophysiological and anatomical data. Pain 82:245–251
13. Ojemann JG, Silbergeld DL (1995) Cortical stimulation mapping of phantom limb rolandic cortex. Case report. J Neurosurg 82: 641–644
14. Penfield W (1975) The physiology of epilepsy. Adv Neurol 8:1–9
15. Roux FE, Lotterie JA, Cassol E, Lazorthes Y, Sol JC, Berry I (2003) Cortical areas involved in virtual movement of phantom limbs: comparison with normal subjects. Neurosurgery 53:1342–1353
16. Saitoh Y, Hirano S, Kato A, Kishima H, Hirata M, Yamamoto K, Yoshimine T (2001) Motor cortex stimulation for deafferentation pain. Neurosurg Focus 11:E1
17. Tsubokawa T, Katayama Y, Yamamoto T, Hirayama T, Koyama S (1993) Chronic motor cortex stimulation in patients with thalamic pain. J Neurosurg 78:393–401
18. Tsubokawa T, Katayama Y, Yamamoto T, Hirayama T, Koyama S (1991) Treatment of thalamic pain by chronic motor cortex stimulation. Pacing Clin Electrophysiol 14:131–134
19. Velasco F, Carrillo-Ruiz JD, Castro G, Argüelles C, Velasco AL, Kassian A, Guevara U (2009) Motor cortex electrical stimulation applied to patients with complex regional pain syndrome. Pain 147:91–98
20. Woolsey CN (1958) Organization of somatic sensory and motor areas of the cerebral cortex. In: Harlow HF, Woolsey CN (eds) Biological and biochemical bases of behavior. University of Wisconsin Press, Madison, pp 63–81
21. Yang TT, Gallen CC, Ramachandran VS, Cobb S, Schwartz BJ, Bloom FE (1994) Noninvasive detection of cerebral plasticity in adult human somatosensory cortex. Neuroreport 5:701–704
22. Yousry TA, Schmid UD, Alkadhi H, Schmidt D, Peraud A, Buettner A, Winkler P (1997) Localization of the motor hand area to a knob on the precentral gyrus. A new landmark. Brain 120:141–157

Restorative Strategies for the Dopaminergic Nigrostriatal Projection Pathway

Guido Nikkhah

Abstract New insights into the mechanism of dopaminergic (DA) nigrostriatal neuron degeneration and regeneration in experimental studies in animal models of Parkinson's disease (PD) have opened up the discussion about novel therapeutic strategies such as cell-based therapies and neuroprotection of DA neurons. These cellular and molecular approaches aim at preventing or slowing down the progressive degeneration of DA neurons and/or replacing the lost ones. Here, a brief overview of basic principles and current strategies of these novel restorative approaches is discussed in light of experimental results and possible clinical applications.

Keywords Parkinson's disease • Fetal and stem cell transplantation • Neuroprotection

Introduction

Parkinson's disease (PD) is characterized by the loss of dopaminergic neurons (DA) in the substantia nigra pars compacta [19] which, in turn, results in pathophysiological changes, with a decrease of the normal nigrostriatal inhibition within the basal ganglia circuitry [45, 48]. Since the basis of the disease is a progressive loss of nigral DA neurons in the substantia nigra, slowing down this pathological process and/or replacing these neurons may significantly attenuate the clinical symptomatology [35]. Demonstrating functional restoration with neural transplantation in PD in the 1980s provided the first evidence for neural repair strategies [30]. In two prospective U.S. studies with sham surgeries as controls during the late 1990s, there was no significant overall clinical benefit. Moreover, some of the patients developed serious dyskinesias. Since those trials used suboptimal methods for cell transplantation and patient selection, such randomised placebo-controlled clinical trials were widely considered as premature [5, 21, 37]. On the other hand, neuroprotective approaches have also progressed from experimental observations towards clinical applications, and are being currently examined in several clinical trials [1, 51]. Since these restorative approaches have the potential to significantly extend the therapeutic armamentarium for PD patients, further investigations in this field are clearly justified and will be discussed.

G. Nikkhah, MD, PhD
Division of Stereotactic and Functional Neurosurgery, Department of General Neurosurgery, Neurosurgical Clinic, University Medical Center Freiburg, Breisacher Straße 64, Freiburg D-79106, Germany

Neurosurgical Clinic, University Hospital Erlangen, Schwabachanlage 6, Erlangen D-91054, Germany
e-mail: guido.nikkhah@uk-erlangen.de

Neural Transplantation

Grafting dopamine-producing cells into different regions of the basal ganglia should compensate, at least partially, for the intrinsic nigrostriatal neuron degeneration seen in PD. Experimental studies in both rodent and primate Parkinson models (Fig. 1) have shown that implanted embryonic dopaminergic neurons survive (Fig. 2), form synaptic connections at the site of implantation, and induce a certain degree of recovery on both sensory and motor deficits [10]. There are a number of critical factors that are now known to determine the extent of functional recovery in the animal model of PD, such as the degree of hemispheric dominance [37], the implantation site and pattern of distribution [12, 39], or mixture between serotonergic and dopaminergic donor cells [15] (for review see also Döbrössy et al. [10]).

Despite the good results obtained by fetal tissue transplantation in these animal experimental models, the first clinical trials in human transplantation were performed with adrenal medullary tissue due to the ethical, immunological, and infectious concerns related to the use of fetal mesencephalic cells [2, 34]. Some authors reported a significant improvement of patient symptoms (rigidity, akinesia, and tremor) after adrenal tissue

DOI 10.1007/978-3-7091-1482-7_13,

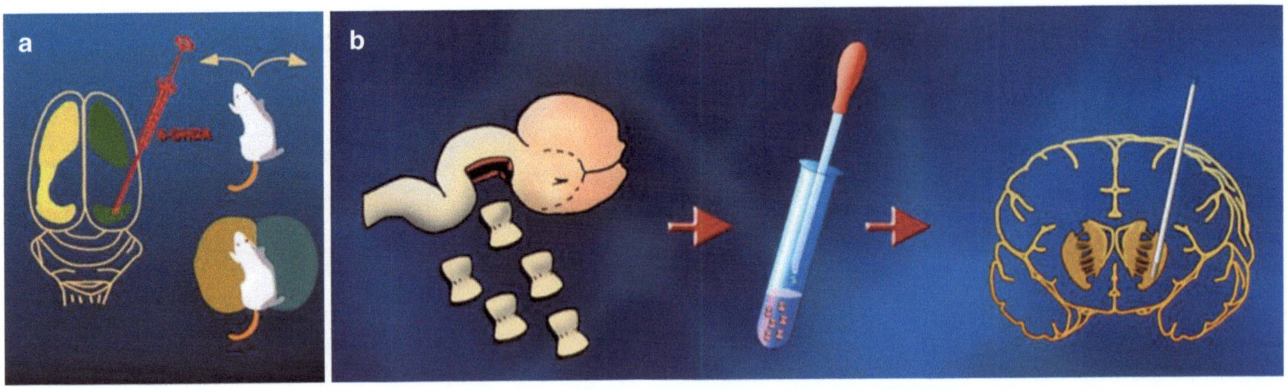

Fig. 1 Schematic diagram representing the (**a**) animal model of PD, which is generated by the unilateral injection of the neurotoxin 6-hydroxydopamine. This leads to a complete unilateral loss of the dopoaminergic innervation concomitant with sensorimotor deficits. (**b**) Shows the individual steps for the grafting procedure. VM tissue is dissected microscopically, mechanically and enzymatically dissociated and, finally, the resulting cell suspension is stereotactically implanted into the striatum

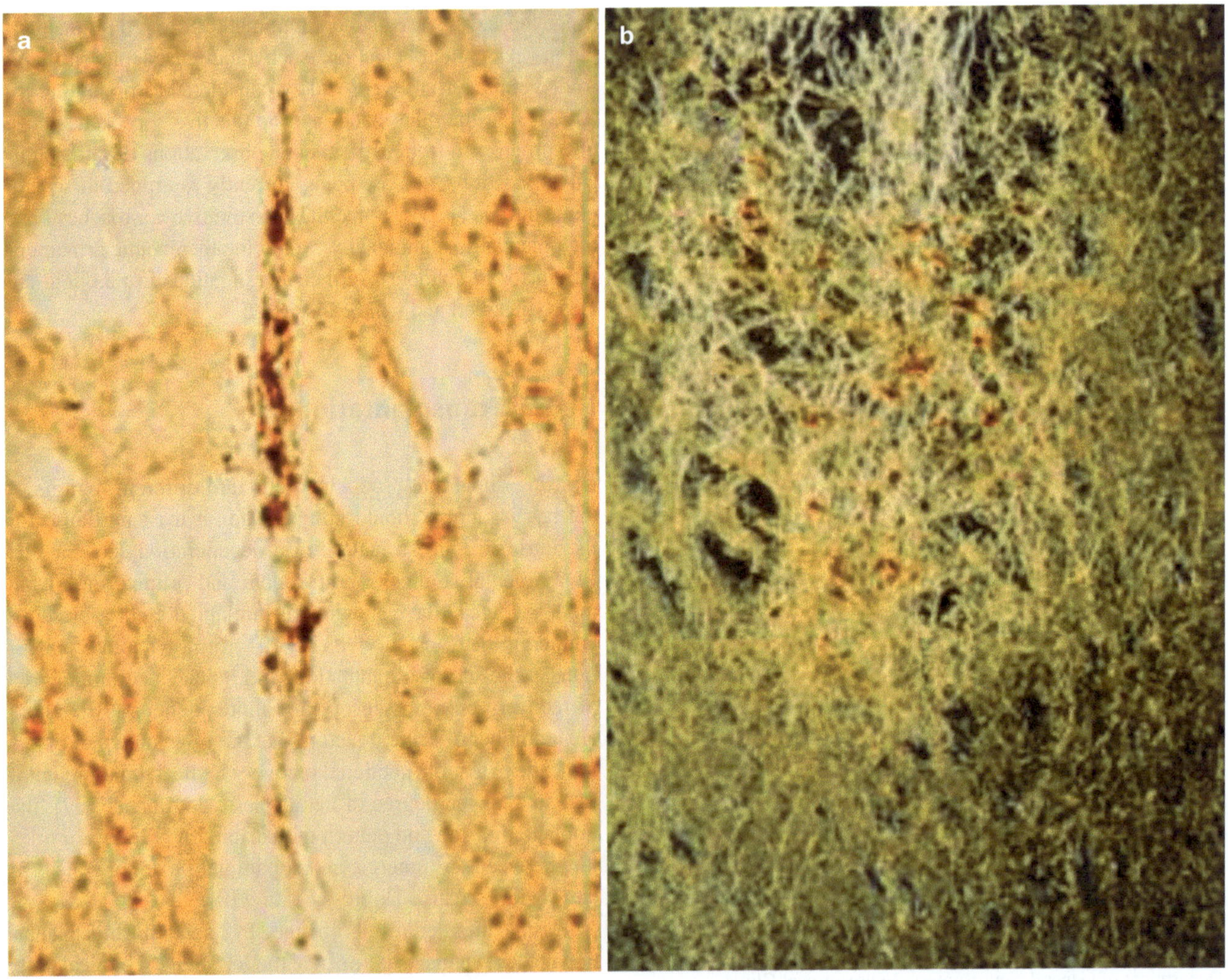

Fig. 2 Dopaminergic graft development in the animal model. A few days after implantation, only small tissue strands are visible (**a**), which expand and develop over the first few weeks into mature grafts reinnervating the surrounding striatum (**b**), as shown by TH-immunohistochemistry

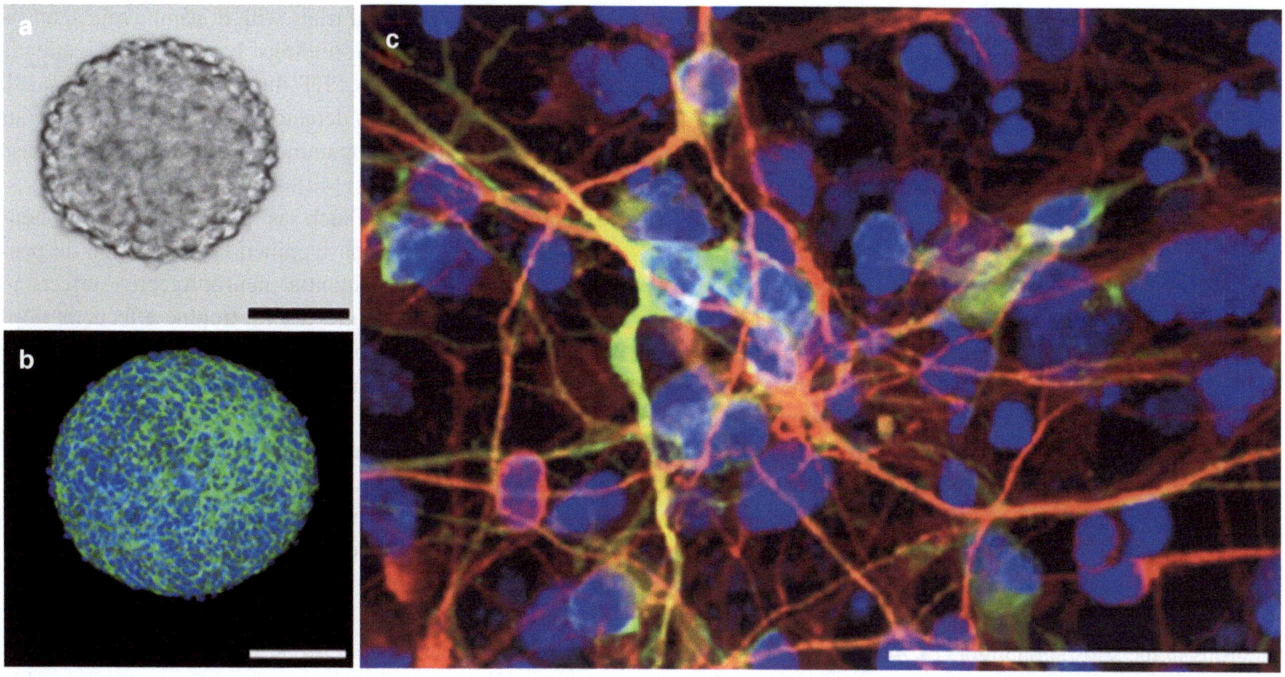

Fig. 3 Neural stem cells (the somatic stem cells of the nervous system) can be propagated as neurosphere cultures applying mitogens such as epidermal growth factor (EGF) and basic fibroblast growth factor (bFGF) for continued expansion. Phase-contrast image of a neurosphere (**a**) derived from human ventral midbrain after long-term expansion (scale bar = 100 μm). Immunostaining shows that neurospheres contain large numbers of nestin-positive cells (**b**) (*green* nestin, *blue* DAPI; scale bar 100 μm). For appropriate differentiation, here into dopaminergic neurons (**c**), a cocktail of patterning factors including brain-derived neurotrophic factor is applied (*green* tyrosine hydroxylase, *red* β-III-tubulin, *blue* DAPI; scale bar = 50 μm) (Modified, from Maciaczyk et al. [33])

grafts or co-grafts (adrenal cells + peripheral nerve) in the caudate nucleus [34]. However, more extensive and critical evaluations revealed only a mild to moderate reduction in "off" time for a limited follow-up period (6–18 months), with no long-term beneficial effects [43]. Therefore, adrenal medullary grafts are not used any longer in clinical practice. Fetal mesencephalic cell transplantation was introduced in clinical trials in 1987, and initial results showed only a moderate improvement during long-term follow up [32]. Optimisation of donor age, number of cells, the use of cell suspensions, and the improvement of stereotactic surgical technique with the use of multiple implantation sites led to a significant improvement in long-term graft survival and graft-induced functional recovery [39, 54].

Fetal mesencephalic cell grafting showed promising positive results, decreasing the patient's time spent in "off", and improving bradykinesia and rigidity as summarized in Winkler et al. 2005 [54]. An increase in "on" time period from 69 to 86 % and improvement of the motor UPDRS scores up to 42 % have been reported after fetal DA transplantation into the caudate and putamen nuclei. Bilateral transplantation of mesencephalic fetal tissue into the putamen showed a significant improvement in the daily life motor and total activities of patients, and additionally an average improvement on the UPDRS score of 32 % over a 2-year follow-up. PET studies displayed an increase of fluorodopa uptake (50–68 %) at the grafting sites up to 6 years after surgery in Parkinson patients. Post-mortem report of two patients, 18 months after neural transplantation surgery, provided clear evidence for good graft survival, axonal outgrowth from the graft cells, and TH-positive reinnervation of the putamen (about 10 %). Interestingly, more recent post-mortem investigations after long-term survival of grafted PD patients have revealed conflicting results with regard to the spreading of PD pathology to grafted cells, despite an overall good survival [24, 29, 36]. In addition, the role of the immunogenicity of grafted fetal neural cells has to be better understood and more carefully addressed in future studies [6].

Still, due to the ethical and methodological limitations implied by the use of human embryonic tissue for transplantation, further progress in this field clearly depends on the successful development of alternative cell resources (Fig. 3), a scientific field which is currently experiencing exciting and promising developments [31, 49, 50].

However, none of these novel alternative cellular resources have yet fully qualified for the initiation of a new clinical trial in PD patients. As basic transplantation research has progressed significantly over recent years, a European-based decision was undertaken to initiate a novel clinical trial using human fetal donor tissue in PD patients. This TransEuro consortium is now actively recruiting patients for a phase I/II clinical transplantation trial which hopefully will set the stage for the prospects of neural grafting in PD in the next few years [11] (see also http://www.transeuro.org.uk/ for further details).

Neuroprotective Therapies

Neuroprotective therapies are aimed on counteracting the different steps and mechanisms involved in the progressive cell degeneration and cell death of nigral dopaminergic neurons in Parkinson's disease. Progressive cell degeneration is most likely due to several different factors, namely oxidative stress, mitochondrial complex I defect, impairment of antioxidant mechanisms (GSH), glutamate excitotoxicity, and electrolyte imbalances (Ca^{2+}, Fe, NO), leading finally to apoptosis and an on-going cell death of the dopaminergic neurons in the substantia nigra [14, 41].

Taking into consideration that in parkinsonian patients a progressive decline on DA cells of about 10 % per year may occur, and that initial symptoms usually appear after a loss of over 50 % of the dopaminergic neurons in the substantia nigra pars compacta, effective neuroprotection treatment could definitively change the natural course of the disease and avoid further clinical deterioration in these patients. Furthermore, PET and spectroscopic computed tomography (SPECT) studies can detect asymptomatic PD patients in the early phases of dopamine degeneration (preclinical PD phase), which could have an enormous impact with regard to the timing for performing such protective approaches.

Many drugs have been used over recent decades in order to rescue or protect the DA nigral neurons from degeneration [42, 44]. Drugs such as pergolide, deprenyl (monoamine oxidase – B inhibitor), and vitamin E (α-Tocopherol) have been investigated in experimental and clinical trials, with the goal of reducing oxidative stress and preserving dopaminergic nigral neurons.

α-Tocopherol has proven to be ineffective as a free radical scavenger for PD [41]. On the other hand, selegiline was able to counteract the progression of PD in experimentally MPTP-induced parkinsonism in animals [44]. However, clinical trials failed to depict any significant effects with regard to a neuroprotection on DA nigral cells and of Parkinson symptoms in a long-term follow-up study [44]. Moreover, complications (hypertension, tachycardia, headache, vomiting) were related with the chronic use of selegiline in high doses [44].

Dopamine agonists have also shown some protective effect in experimental studies [42]. Dopaminergic neurons in culture submitted to different toxins can be protected by using dopamine agonists [42]. Furthermore, 6 – hydroxydopamine (6-OHDA) lesioned rodents and MPTP-primates treated with dopamine agonists have a lower nigral neuronal loss [41, 42]. On the other hand, clinical trials with dopaminergic agonists did not show significant findings based on the patient's UPDRS scores or on the PET flurodopa uptake data [38]. Nevertheless, PET images depicted a positive trend in favour of patients treated with dopamine agonists and short disease duration (less than 2 years) [42].

Neurotrophic factors such as glial cell derived neurotrophic factor (GDNF) have gained large attention for possible treatment and its potential neuroprotective effects in Parkinson patients, due to its strong trophic effects on dopaminergic neurons in vitro and in vivo [22, 55]. Experimental studies in both 6-OHDA rodent and MPTP-primate models of Parkinson's disease have demonstrated preservation or even recovery of dopaminergic cells after intraventricular or intraparenchymal (midbrain) infusion of GDNF [16, 25]. A significant reduction in drug-induced apomorphine rotation and a neuroprotective effect after GDNF infusion into the substantia nigra prior to 6-OHDA lesions in rats have also been reported [22].

In the primate model, a 40 % preservation of DA cells (substantia nigra and putaminal regions) has been reported in animals which received GDNF prior to the MPTP administration compared to 1–7 % in lesioned-only control groups [16]. In these animals, cardinal symptoms like bradykinesia, rigidity, and postural instability have been improved. Nevertheless, the clinical efficacy of GDNF in the treatment of PD or for DA cell neuroprotection in patients with PD has still to be demonstrated [1]. Intraventricular application of GDNF in the first clinical trials failed to show a significant improvement of the main cardinal symptoms of the PD [23].

The Role of the STN in Neuroprotection and the Effects of Glutamate Inhibitors

New insights into the pathophysiology and electrophysiology of the basal ganglia circuitry over recent years led to the discovery of the STN as one of the important targets for surgical treatment in Parkinson's disease [8, 26, 28]. Reduced activity of the afferent inhibitory inputs to the STN due to the degeneration of the nigral dopaminergic neurons leads to STN overactivity and an important glutaminergic excitatory effect on different output structures, which may be an important trigger for the appearance of parkinsonian symptoms [13, 20]. Furthermore, increases in glutamate release may additionally induce and/or sustain SNc dopaminergic neuronal degeneration by cellular Ca^{2+} influx, free radical formation (NO), and intracellular swelling [40]. Based on this excitotoxic hypothesis of glutamate-mediated neuronal cell dysfunction and degeneration, different pharmacological and surgical strategies have been developed in order to rescue DA neurons of the pars compacta of the substantia nigra

(SNc) from further progressive degeneration [9, 40]. Glutamate receptors antagonists have resulted in a neuroprotective effect in DA cell cultures [9]. Electrophysiological experimental analysis in the primate models of PD has shown that release of glutamate influence the neuronal firing rate in the SNc [52, 53]. Administration of NMDA receptor agonists increases substantially the burst activity in the SNc, and application of NMDA antagonists lowers the SNc electrical activity by blocking glutamate effects, which may attenuate the progressive neuronal cell loss [40, 46].

Unfortunately, clinical use may cause serious neuropsychiatric side-effects [46]. Antiglutamate agents that reduce glutamate release have been demonstrated experimentally to exhibit a neuroprotective effect, but this must still be further elucidated [46].

Experimental lesions of the STN have been performed in both non-human primates and in rodent Parkinson models, in order to evaluate the effects on the transneuronal degeneration and progressive loss of dopaminergic cells in the SNc following DA-depleting lesions [46]. Unilateral 6-OHDA-induced axon terminal intrastriatal lesions resulted in a marked loss of TH-positive fiber innervation in the striatum and a substantial degeneration on the SNc dopaminergic neurons [47]. In animals with combined STN and striatal 6-OHDA DA lesions, degeneration of the dopaminergic substantia nigra (SN) neurons was considerably reduced [7].

In monkeys, unilateral STN lesions have been shown to improve the cardinal parkinsonian symptoms such as bradykinesia, akinesia, tremor and, in a less dramatic way, rigidity [3]. In animals in which the STN lesions have been done prior to MPTP injections, drug-induced PD failed to develop, as was observed in control animals, indicating the possibility of a neuroprotective effect in this chronic animal model [3, 46].

More recently, gene transfer-mediated expression of glutamatergic acid decarboxylase (GAD) to modulate GABA production in the STN has shown promising results after 6 months in a clinical trial [27].

Conclusions

Several experimental studies have provided evidence for the role of oxidative stress with the formation of free radicals, the decrease of normal antioxidant defences such as GSH, the defect in the complex I in the mitochondrial respiratory chain, and the importance of glutamate neurotoxicity, among other factors, in the pathophysiology of nigrostriatal dopaminergic cell death [48]. Recently, the pathophysiological role and clinical implication of the STN has received considerable attention. Hyperactivity of the STN in PD, and thus over-secretion of glutamate, may lead to cellular membrane impairment, with an increase of Ca^{+} influx into the cells, activating a cascade of cellular alterations, leading finally to apoptosis and cell death [4]. However, the exact mechanism of action of glutamate-inducing neuronal cell death is still not completely understood. Experimental studies elucidating the exact mechanism of glutamate neurotoxicity and the role of glutamate receptors in the alteration of cellular membrane function could open new frontiers on the therapy and prevention of progressive nigrostriatal dopaminergic degeneration in PD patients. With regard to the effects of STN ablations in animals models of PD, different reports on studies in both rodent and primate models have demonstrated promising results with respect to the recovery of parkinsonian deficits and major symptoms (Bermann; Wichmann III). Unilateral lesions of the STN seems to be well-tolerated by the animals, or cause minimal dyskinetic symptoms which do not significantly impair the normal daily activities in these animals [17]. Clinical trials on lesioning the STN have been rarely performed up to now. First reports from Guridi and Obeso [18] showed a potential recovery of parkinsonian symptoms in a limited number of patients, with low incidence of postoperative complications [18]. Unilateral STN lesions, with precise intraoperative electrophysiological localization, could probably be one surgical alternative for the treatment for Parkinson patients with medically uncontrollable freezing and tremor.

Experimental lesions of the STN have been shown to induce a neuroprotective effect on dopaminergic neurons of the SNc [7]. STN ablations, when performed prior to terminal intrastriatal 6-OHDA lesions in the rodent model for PD, do indeed induce a significant rescue of dopaminergic nigral neurons. However, neuroprotective effects of STN lesions should still be examined in primates, before possible applications in clinical trials in humans. Moreover, unilateral and bilateral deep brain stimulation of the STN, which seems to work as a functional blockade of STN neurons through high-frequency stimulation, have been already shown to induce a significant improvement of major parkinsonian symptoms in patients suffering from severe PD. Based on the neuroprotective findings from experimental STN ablations in animal models, novel mechanisms of actions may now be considered with regard to the potential neuroprotective effects induced by DBS of the STN. However, there is very little experimental or clinical evidence so far. Experimental evaluation of the neuroprotective effect induced by DBS on the STN could, for example, be performed in the MPTP-primate model of PD.

Taken together, novel approaches towards a neuroprotection of dopaminergic neurons by STN lesions or DBS and new cell replacement strategies may add a significant armamentarium to the current neurosurgical treatment options available for patients with Parkinson's disease [35]. Further substantial experimental work has to be carried out for a better understanding of, for example, glutamatergic neurotoxicity, protective effects of STN ablation and DBS, and alternative cell resources for transplantation, in order to provide a profound scientific and ethical basis for the successful development of these new experimental concepts into clinical applications in PD, and potentially also in other neurological disorders.

Acknowledgments Parts of the work presented here have been supported by grants from the Deutsche Forschungsgemeinschaft (Ni 330), the Graduate School Freiburg (DFG 843), the Weber Petri Foundation, the German Parkinson Foundation and the European Commission under the 7th Framework Programme — HEALTH — Collaborative Project Transeuro (Contract n 242003).

Conflict of Interest No potential conflict of interest relevant to this article was reported.

References

1. Aron L, Klein R (2011) Repairing the parkinsonian brain with neurotrophic factors. Trends Neurosci 34:88–100
2. Backlund EO, Granberg PO, Hamberger B, Knutsson E, Martensson A, Sedvall G, Seiger A, Olson L (1985) Transplantation of adrenal medullary tissue to striatum in parkinsonism. First clinical trials. J Neurosurg 62:169–173
3. Bergman H, Wichmann T, DeLong MR (1990) Reversal of experimental parkinsonism by lesions of the subthalamic nucleus. Science 249:1436–1438
4. Blandini F, Porter RH, Greenamyre JT (1996) Glutamate and Parkinson's disease. Mol Neurobiol 12:73–94
5. Brundin P, Dunnett S, Bjorklund A, Nikkhah G (2001) Transplanted dopaminergic neurons: more or less? Nat Med 7:512–513
6. Capetian P, Döbrössy M, Winkler C, Prinz M, Nikkhah G (2011) To be or not to be accepted: the role of immunogenicity of neural stem cells following transplantation into the brain in animal and human studies. Semin Immunopathol 33:619–626
7. Carvalho GA, Nikkhah G (2001) Subthalamic nucleus lesions are neuroprotective against terminal 6-OHDA-induced striatal lesions and restore postural balancing reactions. Exp Neurol 171:405–417
8. Chevalier G, Deniau JM (1990) Disinhibition as a basic process in the expression of striatal functions. Trends Neurosci 13:277–280
9. Choi DW, Rothman SM (1990) The role of glutamate neurotoxicity in hypoxic-ischemic neuronal death. Annu Rev Neurosci 13: 171–182
10. Döbrössy M, Busse M, Piroth T, Rosser A, Dunnett S, Nikkhah G (2010) Neurorehabilitation with neural transplantation. Neurorehabil Neural Repair 24:692–701
11. Dyson SC, Barker RA (2011) Cell-based therapies for Parkinson's disease. Expert Rev Neurother 11:831–844
12. Falkenstein G, Rosenthal C, Reum T, Morgenstern R, Döbrössy M, Nikkhah G (2009) Pattern of long-term sensorimotor recovery following intrastriatal and – accumbens DA micrografts in a rat model of Parkinson's disease. J Comp Neurol 515:41–55
13. Feger J, Hassani OK, Mouroux M (1997) The subthalamic nucleus and its connections. New electrophysiological and pharmacological data. Adv Neurol 74:31–43
14. Foley P, Riederer P (1999) Pathogenesis and preclinical course of Parkinson's disease. J Neural Transm Suppl 56:31–74
15. García J, Carlsson T, Döbrössy M, Nikkhah G, Winkler C (2011) Impact of dopamine to serotonin cell ratio in transplants on behavioral recovery and L-DOPA-induced dyskinesia. Neurobiol Dis 43:576–587
16. Gash DM, Zhang Z, Gerhardt G (1998) Neuroprotective and neurorestorative properties of GDNF. Ann Neurol 44:S121–S125
17. Guridi J, Herrero MT, Luquin MR, Guillen J, Ruberg M, Laguna J, Vila M, Javoy-Agid F, Agid Y, Hirsch E, Obeso JA (1996) Subthalamotomy in parkinsonian monkeys. Behavioural and biochemical analysis. Brain 119(Pt 5):1717–1727
18. Guridi J, Obeso JA (1997) The role of the subthalamic nucleus in the origin of hemiballism and parkinsonism: new surgical perspectives. Adv Neurol 74:235–247
19. Halliday G, Lees A, Stern M (2011) Milestones in Parkinson's disease – clinical and pathologic features. Mov Dis 26:1015–1021
20. Hassani OK, Mouroux M, Feger J (1996) Increased subthalamic neuronal activity after nigral dopaminergic lesion independent of disinhibition via the globus pallidus. Neuroscience 72:105–115
21. Isacson O (2009) Cell therapy ahead for Parkinson's disease. Science 326:1060
22. Kearns CM, Cass WA, Smoot K, Kryscio R, Gash DM (1997) GDNF protection against 6-OHDA: time dependence and requirement for protein synthesis. J Neurosci 17:7111–7118
23. Koller W, Wilkinson S, Pahwa R et al (1998) Surgical treatment options in Parkinson's disease. In: Bakay R (ed) Neurosurgery clinics of North America: surgical treatment movement disorders. W. B. Saunders Company, Philadelphia, pp 295–306
24. Kordower JH, Chu Y, Hauser RA, Freeman TB, Olanow CW (2008) Lewy body-like pathology in long-term embryonic nigral transplants in Parkinson's disease. Nat Med 14(5):504–506
25. Kordower JH, Emborg ME, Bloch J, Ma SY, Chu Y, Leventhal L, McBride J, Chen EY, Palfi S, Roitberg BZ, Brown WD, Holden JE, Pyzalski R, Taylor MD, Carvey P, Ling Z, Trono D, Hantraye P, Deglon N, Aebischer P (2000) Neurodegeneration prevented by lentiviral vector delivery of GDNF in primate models of Parkinson's disease. Science 290:767–773
26. Lang AE, Lozano AM (1998) Parkinson's disease. Second of two parts. N Engl J Med 339:1130–1143
27. LeWitt PA, Rezai AR, Leehey MA, Ojemann SG, Flaherty AW, Eskandar EN, Kostyk SK, Thomas K, Sarkar A, Siddiqui MS, Tatter SB, Schwalb JM, Poston KL, Henderson JM, Kurlan RM, Richard IH, Van Meter L, Sapan CV, During MJ, Kaplitt MG, Feigin A (2011) AAV2-GAD gene therapy for advanced Parkinson's disease: a double-blind, sham-surgery controlled, randomised trial. Lancet Neurol 10:309–319
28. Levy R, Hazrati LN, Herrero MT, Vila M, Hassani OK, Mouroux M, Ruberg M, Asensi H, Agid Y, Feger J, Obeso JA, Parent A, Hirsch EC (1997) Re-evaluation of the functional anatomy of the basal ganglia in normal and Parkinsonian states. Neuroscience 76:335–343
29. Li JY, Englund E, Holton JL, Soulet D, Hagell P, Lees AJ, Lashley T, Quinn NP, Rehncrona S, Bjorklund A, Widner H, Revesz T, Lindvall O, Brundin P (2008) Lewy bodies in grafted neurons in subjects with Parkinson's disease suggest host-to-graft disease propagation. Nat Med 14:501–503
30. Lindvall O, Björklund A (2011) Cell therapeutics in Parkinson's disease. Neurotherapeutics 8:539–548
31. Lindvall O, Kokaia Z (2010) Stem cells in human neurodegenerative disorders – time for clinical translation? J Clin Invest 120:29–40
32. Lindvall O, Rehncrona S, Brundin P, Gustavii B, Astedt B, Widner H, Lindholm T, Bjorklund A, Leenders KL, Rothwell JC, Frackowiak R, Marsden D, Johnels B, Steg G, Freedman R, Hoffer BJ, Seiger A, Bygdeman M, Strömberg I, Olson L (1989) Human fetal dopamine neurons grafted into the striatum in two patients with severe Parkinson's disease. A detailed account of methodology and a 6-month follow-up. Arch Neurol 46:615–631
33. Maciaczyk J, Singec I, Maciaczyk D, Nikkhah G (2008) Combined use of BDNF, ascorbic acid, low oxygen, and prolonged differentiation time generates tyrosine hydroxylase-expressing neurons after long-term in vitro expansion of human fetal midbrain precursor cells. Exp Neurol 213(2):354–362

34. Madrazo I, Drucker-Colin R, Diaz V, Martinez-Mata J, Torres C, Becerril JJ (1987) Open microsurgical autograft of adrenal medulla to the right caudate nucleus in two patients with intractable Parkinson's disease. N Engl J Med 316:831–834
35. Meissner WG, Frasier M, Gasser T, Goetz CG, Lozano A, Piccini P, Obeso JA, Rascol O, Schapira A, Voon V, Weiner DM, Tison F, Bezard E (2011) Priorities in Parkinson's disease research. Nat Rev Drug Discov 10:377–393
36. Mendez I, Vinuela A, Astradsson A, Mukhida K, Hallett P, Robertson H, Tierney T, Holness R, Dagher A, Trojanowski JQ, Isacson O (2008) Dopamine neurons implanted into people with Parkinson's disease survive without pathology for 14 years. Nat Med 14:507–509
37. Nikkhah G (2001) Transplantation of embryonic dopamine neurons for severe Parkinson's disease: potential and pitfalls. Brain Res Bull 56:509
38. Nikkhah G, Falkenstein G, Rosenthal C (2001) Restorative plasticity of dopamine neuronal transplants depends on the degree of hemispheric dominance. J Neurosci 21:6252–6263
39. Nikkhah G, Rosenthal C, Falkenstein G, Roedter A, Papazoglou A, Brandis A (2009) Microtransplantation of dopaminergic cell suspensions: further characterization and optimization of grafting parameters. Cell Transplant 18:119–133
40. Novelli A, Reilly JA, Lysko PG, Henneberry RC (1988) Glutamate becomes neurotoxic via the N-methyl-D-aspartate receptor when intracellular energy levels are reduced. Brain Res 451:205–212
41. Olanow CW (1997) Attempts to obtain neuroprotection in Parkinson's disease. Neurology 49:S26–S33
42. Olanow CW, Jenner P, Brooks D (1998) Dopamine agonists and neuroprotection in Parkinson's disease. Ann Neurol 44:S167–S174
43. Olanow CW, Koller W, Goetz CG, Stebbins GT, Cahill DW, Gauger LL, Morantz R, Penn RD, Tanner CM, Klawans HL, Shannon KM, Comella CL, Witt T (1990) Autologous transplantation of adrenal medulla in Parkinson's disease. 18-month results. Arch Neurol 47:1286–1289
44. Olanow CW, Mytilineou C, Tatton W (1998) Current status of selegiline as a neuroprotective agent in Parkinson's disease. Mov Disord 13(Suppl 1):55–58
45. Quinn N (1997) Parkinson's disease: clinical features. In: Quinn N (ed) Clinical neurology. Parkinsonism. Bailliere Tindall, London, pp 1–13
46. Rodriguez MC, Obeso JA, Olanow CW (1998) Subthalamic nucleus-mediated excitotoxicity in Parkinson's disease: a target for neuroprotection. Ann Neurol 44:S175–S188
47. Roedter A, Winkler C, Samii M, Nikkhah G (2000) Complex sensorimotor behavioral changes after terminal striatal 6-OHDA lesion and transplantation of dopaminergic embryonic micrografts. Cell Transplant 9:197–214
48. Schapira A (1997) Pathogenesis of Parkinson's disease. In: Quinn N (ed) Clinical neurology. International practice and research. Parkinsonism. Bailliere Tindall, London, pp 15–36
49. Singec I, Jandial R, Crain A, Nikkhah G, Snyder EY (2007) The leading edge of stem cell therapeutics. Annu Rev Med 58: 313–328
50. Singec I, Knoth R, Meyer RP, Maciaczyk J, Volk B, Nikkhah G, Frotscher M, Snyder EY (2006) Defining the actual sensitivity and specificity of the neurosphere assay in stem cell biology. Nat Methods 3:801–806
51. Smith GS, Laxton AW, Tang-Wai DF, McAndrews MP, Diaconescu AO, Workman CI, Lozano AM (2012) Increased cerebral metabolism after 1 year of deep brain stimulation in Alzheimer disease. Arch Neurol. doi:10.1001/archneurol.2012.590
52. Wichmann T, Bergman H, DeLong MR (1994) The primate subthalamic nucleus. I. Functional properties in intact animals. J Neurophysiol 72:494–506
53. Wichmann T, Bergman H, DeLong MR (1994) The primate subthalamic nucleus. III. Changes in motor behavior and neuronal activity in the internal pallidum induced by subthalamic inactivation in the MPTP model of parkinsonism. J Neurophysiol 72:521–530
54. Winkler C, Kirik D, Bjorklund A (2005) Cell transplantation in Parkinson's disease: how can we make it work? Trends Neurosci 28:86–92
55. Winkler C, Sauer H, Lee CS, Björklund A (1996) Short-term GDNF treatment provides long-term rescue of lesioned nigral dopamine neurons in a rat model of Parkinson's disease. J Neurosci 16: 7206–7215

Some Recent Trends and Further Promising Directions in Functional Neurosurgery

Travis S. Tierney, Tejas Sankar, and Andres M. Lozano

Abstract The field of functional neurosurgery has developed a number of recent innovative neuromodulatory approaches to treat disease that remains resistant to the best medical therapy. These include novel surgical techniques to intervene in motor and cognitive sequelae of refractory epilepsy, neurodegenerative disease, and certain psychiatric conditions. To a large extent, much of the innovation in our field continues to be driven by a systems-level understanding of the impact of disease on the brain. For example, several groups have exploited findings from neuroimaging work to identify a number of new potential neuromodulatory targets for the treatment of refractory depression. Ongoing discoveries at the cellular and molecular level promise targeted gene or drug delivery aimed at curing disease. Neurosurgeons will certainly remain at the forefront of translating these strategies into practical clinical applications. Several randomized trials are now underway to assess the safety and efficacy of a number of new approaches, and we will continue to acquire better knowledge of optimal patient selection, identification of the most effective neuromodulatory targets, and recognition of adverse effects as these studies progress.

T.S. Tierney, MD, PhD
Department of Neurosurgery, Brigham and Women's Hospital, Harvard Medical School, 75 Francis Street, Boston, MA 02115, USA

T. Sankar, MDCM
Division of Neurosurgery, Toronto Western Hospital, 399 Bathurst Street, Toronto, ON M5T 2S8, Canada

A.M. Lozano, MD, PhD, FRCSC, FRS (✉)
Division of Neurosurgery, Toronto Western Hospital, 399 Bathurst Street, Toronto, ON M5T 2S8, Canada

Department of Neurosurgery, University of Toronto, Toronto Western Hospital, 399 Bathurst Street, WW 4-431, Toronto, ON M5T 2S8, Canada
e-mail: lozano@uhnres.utoronto.ca

Keywords Alzheimer's disease • Epilepsy • Deep brain stimulation • Huntington's disease • Depression • Gene therapy • Parkinson's disease • Pedunculopontine nucleus

Introduction

Current trends and new directions in the field of functional neurosurgery are being driven by an increased understanding of the pathophysiological basis of refractory disease in psychiatry and neurology. Indeed, neurosurgeons are once again beginning to treat disease previously considered to be best managed by pharmacological therapy. We review here key emerging neuromodulatory indications for refractory epilepsy, neurodegenerative disease, and certain psychiatric conditions. Evidence for effective and safe surgical intervention in these areas comes from a number of recent clinical trials. We close with a few thoughts on some of the more promising potential directions in functional neurosurgery.

Refractory Epilepsy

Several targets have been suggested for the treatment of medically intractable epilepsy, including stimulation of the cerebral cortex, thalamus, hippocampus, caudate nucleus, locus coeruleus, subthalamic nucleus, and vagus nerve. Two approaches have been assessed in well-known randomized multi-center trials: vagal nerve stimulation and thalamic anterior nucleus deep brain stimulation (DBS). Based on two trials conducted in the mid-1990s, the Food and Drug Administration (FDA) approved vagal nerve stimulation for treatment refractory epilepsy in 1997 [25, 60]. However, seizure control in these studies was quite modest, with only a third of the patents experiencing

DOI 10.1007/978-3-7091-1482-7_14,

at least a 50 % reduction in seizure frequency. Virtually none of these patients were made seizure-free. More recently, the SANTE (Stimulation of Anterior Nucleus of the Thalamus for Epilepsy) trial enrolled 110 adults with partial or generalized seizures unamenable to conventional ablative surgery [17]. Each patient underwent bilateral implantation of standard quadripolar DBS electrodes into the anterior nucleus of the thalamus. Half received 3 months of continuous high-frequency stimulation; the control half were also implanted but not stimulated. At the end of the 3-month pilot period, the stimulated group experienced a 29 % greater reduction in seizures compared with unstimulated controls. All patients in the study then went on to receive unblinded stimulation for 2 years. At the completion of the trial, overall median reduction in seizure frequency was 56 %. More than half of the patients enrolled benefited from seizure reductions of at least 50 %, and 14 patients were completely seizure-free. Based on these findings, the Neurological Devices Advisory Panel of the Food and Drug Administration (FDA) voted to recommend approval of anterior nucleus stimulation as an adjunctive therapy for adult patients with severe refractory epilepsy. Final FDA approval is pending.

Another neuromodulatory approach to the treatment of epilepsy is closed-loop detection of epileptiform activity combined with intermittent cortical intracranial stimulation [53, 55]. This approach is designed to deliver abortive stimulation to the penumbra of epileptic foci only when early discharges are detected; as such, its primary application is in the treatment of discrete epileptic foci within eloquent areas. The results of the first controlled trial of responsive cortical stimulation for medically intractable partial epilepsy have recently been published [45]. The authors reported a statistically significant—though relatively mild—reduction in seizure frequency in active versus sham stimulation groups (37.9 % versus 17.3 % respectively) during the initial blinded phase of the study. Patients who were initially in the sham group showed further improvement once they began to receive active stimulation during the open-label phase, and responsive stimulation was generally well-tolerated across all patients.

It is clear from all of these trials that a substantial fraction of patients received little benefit from invasive stimulation. On the other hand, these studies also show that non-ablative neuromodulation for refractory epilepsy carries quite favorable surgical morbidity and is, in some cases, entirely reversible. More studies are needed, particularly in children, to determine optimal anatomical or electrophysiological predictors of excellent post-operative outcomes.

Parkinson's Disease

Although a number of recent large clinical trials have established the safety and efficacy of pallidal and subthalamic stimulation for the treatment of Parkinson's disease [1, 9, 61, 62], these standard targets do little to relieve the gait and postural disturbance that is often associated with advanced disease [57]. Falls are a major driver of morbidity in this population, conferring a significant risk of head trauma and hip fracture [31]. This observation has prompted a search for other neuromodulatory targets that may improve these and other so-called dopamine non-responsive symptoms that are refractory to both standard levodopa therapy and current surgical interventions [51, 58].

A new indication for an established neuromodulatory intervention was recently suggested by a study of dorsal column stimulation in a rat model of Parkinson's disease, where cervical epidural electrodes were shown to disrupt low-frequency (beta) oscillation between the cortex and striatum with a significant associated improvement in locomotor function [18]. Although initial clinical experience with spinal cord stimulation in patients with Parkinson's disease has been disappointing [56], further work to define optimal patient selection criteria, electrode placement, and effective stimulation parameters may yet yield an effective niche for this relatively safe intervention. Another neuromodulatory target clearly emerging as an effective surgical treatment for medication-resistant locomotor dysfunction is low-frequency stimulation of the pedunculopontine nuclear complex (PPN) [48]. Using standard quadripolar electrodes, several groups have shown in open label trials that PPN DBS is capable of decreasing the frequency of gait freezing and reducing the tendency to fall [16, 42, 43, 49, 54]. However, there are still a number of outstanding issues that require further investigation, including the precise target of electrical stimulation with the PPN region, selection of best responders, and durability of the intervention. Long-term controlled trials of PPN stimulation are being designed to address these questions.

Alzheimer's Disease

Compared with Parkinson's disease, the sociomedical burden of the most common neurodegenerative disease is probably many times greater. Alzheimer's disease currently affects over 27 million people worldwide, and its prevalence will continue to increase as world population ages [4]. Based on an unexpected clinical observation [23], our group initiated a phase I trial of bilateral forniceal stimulation aimed at improving working memory and cognitive function in six patients with Alzheimer's disease. Initial results are encouraging [32]. After 1 year of continuous high-frequency stimulation, the average rate of cognitive decline appears to have been delayed, with significant activation of many memory-associated cortical and subcortical areas, including the hippocampus and entorhinal cortex (Fig. 1). No significant adverse effects on sleep, weight loss, or endocrine function were detected. These findings have led to the organization of a large multi-center trial designed to establish the efficacy of forniceal stimulation when combined with standard pharmacological therapy.

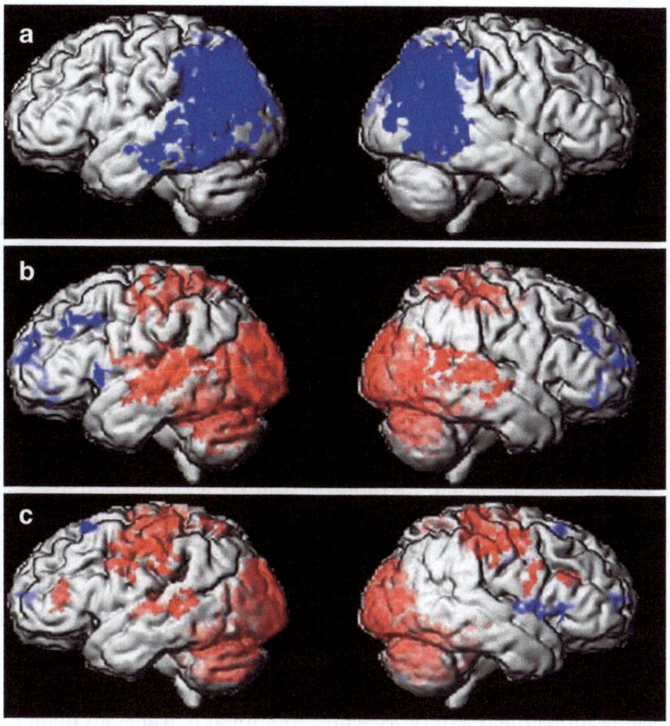

Fig. 1 [^{18}F]-FDG PET scans to measure cerebral glucose metabolism at baseline (**a**), 1 month (**b**) and 1 year (**c**) after deep brain stimulation of the fornix in a single patient with Alzheimer's disease. *Blue* represents areas of decreased glucose uptake, and *red* shows areas of increase glucose utilization between conditions noted on the *right*. After 1 year of chronic high-frequency stimulation, glucose hypometabolic uptake within the temporoparietal cortex that is characteristic of the diseased brain shown in panel **a** was largely reversed as shown in panel **c** (Used with permission from Laxton et al. [32])

Huntington's Disease

Case reports have suggested that lesions of the pallidum may effectively reduce the severity of chorea in patients with chorea-acanthocytosis [19] or Huntington's disease [59]. On the basis of these reports, the possibility of surgically palliating the intractable hyperkinetic movements associated with Huntington's using chronic pallidal stimulation is now being explored. Initial results from six case reports confirm significant reductions in chorea (39–77 %) following bilateral DBS targeting the posteroventral pallidum [2, 13, 26, 28, 44]. As with DBS in dystonia and Parkinson's disease, high-frequency stimulation (130–180 Hz) appears to be optimal, though some authors report that it may worsen bradykinesia and suggest instead that 40 Hz stimulation may be maximally efficacious [13]. To date, there are no data to make the case that stimulation has any effect against the cognitive and behavioural manifestations of the disease. Moving forward, larger case series will be necessary to avoid problems with positive selection bias, refine patient selection criteria, determine the optimal stimulation settings, and establish the long-term efficacy of DBS in this devastating condition.

Treatment-Resistant Depression

Surgical intervention is once more being considered for a number of medically-refractory psychiatric conditions. Clinicians and patients have become increasingly familiar with the limits of pharmacological therapies used to treat many Axis I disorders. This, coupled with significant strides in unraveling the pathophysiological bases of several of these disorders, has led to renewed interest in surgical treatment for many of these conditions. Among the most successful indications for invasive psychiatric neuromodulation has been high-frequency stimulation of limbic circuits for intractable depression. Worldwide, more than 121 million people currently fulfill DSM-4 criteria for major depression [63]. Because 10–20 % of patients treated for major depression fail standard medical, cognitive, and electroconvulsive therapies [8, 14], there is an urgent need for effective new therapy. Currently, several targets for DBS are being investigated for the treatment of intractable major depression, including the subcallosal cingulum, the inferior thalamic peduncle, the nucleus accumbens, and the anterior limb of the internal capsule. The largest number of patients (about 100) have undergone chronic high-frequency stimulation of cingulate white matter tracts near Brodmann area 25. The rationale for targeting this area is derived from PET imaging studies of patients with major depression, demonstrating increased blood flow in that region and decreased flow in associated prefrontal cortical areas [40, 52]. This pattern of activation in depressed patients is largely reversed after successful treatment with antidepressants, cognitive behavioral therapy, or electroconvulsive therapy [10, 21, 39, 47]. Based on these observations, we undertook continuous high-frequency stimulation of the subcallosal cingulate region in patients with treatment-resistant depression [41]. Over 60 % of such patients responded to this intervention, and a third were in complete remission at 6 months. After 1, 3, and

6 years of follow-up, these effects appear to be well-maintained [30, 37]. Two recent prospective, open-label trials of subcallosal cingulate stimulation [27, 36], including one with a sham lead-in phase [27], have largely confirmed these results.

Gene Therapy and Optogenetics

Many of the above conditions have been shown to have clear genetic contributions, and gene therapy may ultimately hold the best hope for a number of chronic neurological conditions. Already in Parkinson's disease, for example, many innovative and potentially effective gene-based therapies seem to be on the horizon. An interesting approach using glutamic acid decarboxylase gene-constructs delivered via an adeno-associated viral vector is being used to convert subthalamic nucleus neurons to an inhibitory phenotype [11, 15], with the intent to reduce excitatory overactivity that is thought to be a central driver of basal ganglia dysfunction. Preliminary clinical trials have demonstrated safety as well as some efficacy using this unique approach [29, 33]. Similarly, clinical trials using gene therapy to upregulate key enzymes in the dopamine metabolic pathway have shown promising results [5, 12]. Although several clinical studies of putative neuroprotective agents have been disappointing, the use of neurotrophic gene therapy with Neurturin is being re-examined in a double-blind trial of infusion at multiple sites including the putamen and substantia nigra [20, 38].

Exciting work in the basic neurosciences has shown it is possible to combine gene therapy with light stimulation, using a technique called optogenetics [3, 46, 64]. In these experiments, neurons are transfected with light-sensitive ion channels using targeted viral vector delivery methods [24]. The primary advantage of this approach may be more precise targeting of specific neural elements (neurons versus fibers of passage, for example) and reduced off-target effects sometimes seen with conventional electrical simulation [22].

Ethical Issues in Novel Neuromodulation

As the frontiers for neuromodulation expand to include conditions where patient autonomy and competence may be impaired, treating physicians and research scientists must consider certain ethical principles and follow basic established guidelines to protect individual patients involved in clinical experiments [6, 7, 50]. Many of the conditions discussed in this article render patients vulnerable by causing physical, cognitive, and emotional disabilities, some to the extent that they are not able to provide valid informed consent. Lipsman and colleagues [34] have proposed a set of ethical criteria for clinical trials in psychiatric neurosurgery which are sufficiently generalizable for application to a wide range of experimental indications for deep brain stimulation. These criteria address aspects of patient selection, disease burden, and refractoriness to known therapy, involvement of multidisciplinary research and care teams, provision of dispassionate regulation and oversight, and ongoing evaluation to identify challenges for the ethical conduct of clinical trials. Importantly, a central consideration is that the process of valid informed consent may be compromised in patients who are cognitively or emotionally impaired by their disease [34, 35]. At an extreme is the issue of proxy consent for experimental research on individuals who have limited legal capacity, e.g., the demented, minimally conscious, children and patients with psychosis. A large body of ethical literature, consensus guidelines, and legal safeguards exists to protect these populations. A more common scenario occurs when a competent patient harbors desperately optimistic expectations for an experimental intervention. Here, the process of informed consent must be completely transparent and free of any potential investigator bias. A general solution is the involvement of disinterested third parties at the level of study oversight by ad hoc expert committees, IRB, and independent external reviewers. The primary goal is the production of rigorous unbiased data where any reasonable risk to a research subject is offset by a potential benefit. Only this kind of data will allow us to avoid pitfalls of the past.

Conclusion

The spectrum of disease indications for neuromodulatory intervention is currently undergoing a dramatic expansion. The model paradigm for development of novel surgical therapy in the field of functional neurosurgery can be drawn from the many successful studies designed over the last few decades to advance a more effective treatment for Parkinson's disease. Some of this success may be being translated into better treatments for other neurodegenerative and psychiatric conditions that have also proven resistant to standard medical care. The types of treatments ultimately most useful to patients and their caregivers will be those that most effectively control the behavioral manifestations of the disease. However, deeper understanding of the underlying disease pathology permits investigators to conceive of completely novel approaches that may hold the best hope for a cure.

Conflict of Interest TST and TS declare that they have no conflict of interest. AML holds intellectual property rights in the field of deep brain stimulation, and has served as a consultant for Medtronic and St. Jude corporations.

References

1. Benabid AL, Chabardes S, Seigneuret E (2005) Deep-brain stimulation in Parkinson's disease: long-term efficacy and safety – what happened this year? Curr Opin Neurol 18:623–630
2. Biolsi B, Cif L, Fertit HE, Robles SG, Coubes P (2008) Long-term follow-up of Huntington disease treated by bilateral deep brain stimulation of the internal globus pallidus. J Neurosurg 109: 130–132
3. Boyden ES, Zhang F, Bamberg E, Nagel G, Deisseroth K (2005) Millisecond-timescale, genetically targeted optical control of neural activity. Nat Neurosci 8:1263–1268
4. Brookmeyer R, Johnson E, Ziegler-Graham K, Arrighi HM (2007) Forecasting the global burden of Alzheimer's disease. Alzheimers Dement 3:186–191
5. Christine CW, Starr PA, Larson PS, Eberling JL, Jagust WJ, Hawkins RA, VanBrocklin HF, Wright JF, Bankiewicz KS, Aminoff MJ (2009) Safety and tolerability of putaminal AADC gene therapy for Parkinson disease. Neurology 73:1662–1669
6. Clausen J (2009) Man, machine and in between. Nature 457:1080–1081
7. Clausen J (2010) Ethical brain stimulation – neuroethics of deep brain stimulation in research and clinical practice. Eur J Neurosci 32:1152–1162
8. Depression Guideline Panel (1993) Depression in primary care, vol 2, Treatment of major depression. US Department of Health and Human Services, Agency for Health Care Policy and Research; AHCPR Publication, Rockville
9. Deuschl G, Schade-Brittinger C, Krack P, Volkmann J, Schafer H, Botzel K, Daniels C, Deutschlander A, Dillmann U, Eisner W, Gruber D, Hamel W, Herzog J, Hilker R, Klebe S, Kloss M, Koy J, Krause M, Kupsch A, Lorenz D, Lorenzl S, Mehdorn HM, Moringlane JR, Oertel W, Pinsker MO, Reichmann H, Reuss A, Schneider GH, Schnitzler A, Steude U, Sturm V, Timmermann L, Tronnier V, Trottenberg T, Wojtecki L, Wolf E, Poewe W, Voges J (2006) A randomized trial of deep-brain stimulation for Parkinson's disease. N Engl J Med 355:896–908
10. Dougherty DD, Weiss AP, Cosgrove GR, Alpert NM, Cassem EH, Nierenberg AA, Price BH, Mayberg HS, Fischman AJ, Rauch SL (2003) Cerebral metabolic correlates as potential predictors of response to anterior cingulotomy for treatment of major depression. J Neurosurg 99:1010–1017
11. During MJ, Kaplitt MG, Stern MB, Eidelberg D (2001) Subthalamic GAD gene transfer in Parkinson disease patients who are candidates for deep brain stimulation. Hum Gene Ther 12:1589–1591
12. Eberling JL, Jagust WJ, Christine CW, Starr P, Larson P, Bankiewicz KS, Aminoff MJ (2008) Results from a phase I safety trial of hAADC gene therapy for Parkinson disease. Neurology 70:1980–1983
13. Fasano A, Mazzone P, Piano C, Quaranta D, Soleti F, Bentivoglio AR (2008) GPi-DBS in Huntington's disease: results on motor function and cognition in a 72-year-old case. Mov Disord 23: 1289–1292
14. Fava M (2003) Diagnosis and definition of treatment-resistant depression. Biol Psychiatry 53:649–659
15. Feigin A, Kaplitt MG, Tang C, Lin T, Mattis P, Dhawan V, During MJ, Eidelberg D (2007) Modulation of metabolic brain networks after subthalamic gene therapy for Parkinson's disease. Proc Natl Acad Sci USA 104:19559–19564
16. Ferraye MU, Debu B, Fraix V, Goetz L, Ardouin C, Yelnik J, Henry-Lagrange C, Seigneuret E, Piallat B, Krack P, Le Bas JF, Benabid AL, Chabardes S, Pollak P (2010) Effects of pedunculopontine nucleus area stimulation on gait disorders in Parkinson's disease. Brain 133:205–214
17. Fisher R, Salanova V, Witt T, Worth R, Henry T, Gross R, Oommen K, Osorio I, Nazzaro J, Labar D, Kaplitt M, Sperling M, Sandok E, Neal J, Handforth A, Stern J, DeSalles A, Chung S, Shetter A, Bergen D, Bakay R, Henderson J, French J, Baltuch G, Rosenfeld W, Youkilis A, Marks W, Garcia P, Barbaro N, Fountain N, Bazil C, Goodman R, McKhann G, Babu Krishnamurthy K, Papavassiliou S, Epstein C, Pollard J, Tonder L, Grebin J, Coffey R, Graves N (2010) Electrical stimulation of the anterior nucleus of thalamus for treatment of refractory epilepsy. Epilepsia 51:899–908
18. Fuentes R, Petersson P, Siesser WB, Caron MG, Nicolelis MA (2009) Spinal cord stimulation restores locomotion in animal models of Parkinson's disease. Science 323:1578–1582
19. Fujimoto Y, Isozaki E, Yokochi F, Yamakawa K, Takahashi H, Hirai S (1997) A case of chorea-acanthocytosis successfully treated with posteroventral pallidotomy. Rinsho Shinkeigaku 37:891–894
20. Gasmi M, Herzog CD, Brandon EP, Cunningham JJ, Ramirez GA, Ketchum ET, Bartus RT (2007) Striatal delivery of neurturin by CERE-120, an AAV2 vector for the treatment of dopaminergic neuron degeneration in Parkinson's disease. Mol Ther 15:62–68
21. Goldapple K, Segal Z, Garson C, Lau M, Bieling P, Kennedy S, Mayberg H (2004) Modulation of cortical-limbic pathways in major depression: treatment-specific effects of cognitive behavior therapy. Arch Gen Psychiatry 61:34–41
22. Gradinaru V, Mogri M, Thompson KR, Henderson JM, Deisseroth K (2009) Optical deconstruction of parkinsonian neural circuitry. Science 324:354–359
23. Hamani C, McAndrews MP, Cohn M, Oh M, Zumsteg D, Shapiro CM, Wennberg RA, Lozano AM (2008) Memory enhancement induced by hypothalamic/fornix deep brain stimulation. Ann Neurol 63:119–123
24. Han X, Boyden ES (2007) Multiple-color optical activation, silencing, and desynchronization of neural activity, with single-spike temporal resolution. PLoS One 2:e299
25. Handforth A, DeGiorgio CM, Schachter SC, Uthman BM, Naritoku DK, Tecoma ES, Henry TR, Collins SD, Vaughn BV, Gilmartin RC, Labar DR, Morris GL 3rd, Salinsky MC, Osorio I, Ristanovic RK, Labiner DM, Jones JC, Murphy JV, Ney GC, Wheless JW (1998) Vagus nerve stimulation therapy for partial-onset seizures: a randomized active-control trial. Neurology 51:48–55
26. Hebb MO, Garcia R, Gaudet P, Mendez IM (2006) Bilateral stimulation of the globus pallidus internus to treat choreathetosis in Huntington's disease: technical case report. Neurosurgery 58:E383; discussion E383
27. Holtzheimer PE, Kelley ME, Gross RE, Filkowski MM, Garlow SJ, Barrocas A, Wint D, Craighead MC, Kozarsky J, Chismar R, Moreines JL, Mewes K, Posse PR, Gutman DA, Mayberg HS (2012) Subcallosal cingulate deep brain stimulation for treatment-resistant unipolar and bipolar depression. Arch Gen Psychiatry 69:150–158
28. Kang GA, Heath S, Rothlind J, Starr PA (2011) Long-term follow-up of pallidal deep brain stimulation in two cases of Huntington's disease. J Neurol Neurosurg Psychiatry 82:272–277
29. Kaplitt MG, Feigin A, Tang C, Fitzsimons HL, Mattis P, Lawlor PA, Bland RJ, Young D, Strybing K, Eidelberg D, During MJ (2007) Safety and tolerability of gene therapy with an adeno-associated virus (AAV) borne GAD gene for Parkinson's disease: an open label, phase I trial. Lancet 369:2097–2105
30. Kennedy SH, Giacobbe P, Rizvi SJ, Placenza FM, Nishikawa Y, Mayberg HS, Lozano AM (2011) Deep brain stimulation for treatment-resistant depression: follow-up after 3 to 6 years. Am J Psychiatry 168(5):502–510
31. Kerr GK, Worringham CJ, Cole MH, Lacherez PF, Wood JM, Silburn PA (2010) Predictors of future falls in Parkinson disease. Neurology 75:116–124
32. Laxton AW, Tang-Wai DF, McAndrews MP, Zumsteg D, Wennberg R, Keren R, Wherrett J, Naglie G, Hamani C, Smith GS, Lozano AM (2010) A phase I trial of deep brain stimulation of memory circuits in Alzheimer's disease. Ann Neurol 68:521–534

33. LeWitt PA, Rezai AR, Leehey MA, Ojemann SG, Flaherty AW, Eskandar EN, Kostyk SK, Thomas K, Sarkar A, Siddiqui MS, Tatter SB, Schwalb JM, Poston KL, Henderson JM, Kurlan RM, Richard IH, Van Meter L, Sapan CV, During MJ, Kaplitt MG, Feigin A (2011) AAV2-GAD gene therapy for advanced Parkinson's disease: a double-blind, sham-surgery controlled, randomised trial. Lancet Neurol 10:309–319
34. Lipsman N, Bernstein M, Lozano AM (2010) Criteria for the ethical conduct of psychiatric neurosurgery clinical trials. Neurosurg Focus 29:E9
35. Lipsman N, Giacobbe P, Bernstein M, Lozano AM (2012) Informed consent for clinical trials of deep brain stimulation in psychiatric disease: challenges and implications for trial design. J Med Ethics 38:107–111
36. Lozano AM, Giacobbe P, Hamani C, Rizvi SJ, Kennedy SH, Kolivakis TT, Debonnel G, Sadikot AF, Lam RW, Howard AK, Ilcewicz-Klimek M, Honey CR, Mayberg HS (2012) A multicenter pilot study of subcallosal cingulate area deep brain stimulation for treatment-resistant depression. J Neurosurg 116:315–322
37. Lozano AM, Mayberg HS, Giacobbe P, Hamani C, Craddock RC, Kennedy SH (2008) Subcallosal cingulate gyrus deep brain stimulation for treatment-resistant depression. Biol Psychiatry 64:461–467
38. Marks WJ Jr, Ostrem JL, Verhagen L, Starr PA, Larson PS, Bakay RA, Taylor R, Cahn-Weiner DA, Stoessl AJ, Olanow CW, Bartus RT (2008) Safety and tolerability of intraputaminal delivery of CERE-120 (adeno-associated virus serotype 2-neurturin) to patients with idiopathic Parkinson's disease: an open-label, phase I trial. Lancet Neurol 7:400–408
39. Mayberg HS, Brannan SK, Tekell JL, Silva JA, Mahurin RK, McGinnis S, Jerabek PA (2000) Regional metabolic effects of fluoxetine in major depression: serial changes and relationship to clinical response. Biol Psychiatry 48:830–843
40. Mayberg HS, Liotti M, Brannan SK, McGinnis S, Mahurin RK, Jerabek PA, Silva JA, Tekell JL, Martin CC, Lancaster JL, Fox PT (1999) Reciprocal limbic-cortical function and negative mood: converging PET findings in depression and normal sadness. Am J Psychiatry 156:675–682
41. Mayberg HS, Lozano AM, Voon V, McNeely HE, Seminowicz D, Hamani C, Schwalb JM, Kennedy SH (2005) Deep brain stimulation for treatment-resistant depression. Neuron 45:651–660
42. Mazzone P, Sposato S, Insola A, Dilazzaro V, Scarnati E (2008) Stereotactic surgery of nucleus tegmenti pedunculopontine [corrected]. Br J Neurosurg 22(Suppl 1):S33–S40
43. Moro E, Hamani C, Poon YY, Al-Khairallah T, Dostrovsky JO, Hutchison WD, Lozano AM (2010) Unilateral pedunculopontine stimulation improves falls in Parkinson's disease. Brain 133:215–224
44. Moro E, Lang AE, Strafella AP, Poon YY, Arango PM, Dagher A, Hutchison WD, Lozano AM (2004) Bilateral globus pallidus stimulation for Huntington's disease. Ann Neurol 56:290–294
45. Morrell MJ (2011) Responsive cortical stimulation for the treatment of medically intractable partial epilepsy. Neurology 77:1295–1304
46. Nagel G, Ollig D, Fuhrmann M, Kateriya S, Musti AM, Bamberg E, Hegemann P (2002) Channelrhodopsin-1: a light-gated proton channel in green algae. Science 296:2395–2398
47. Nobler MS, Oquendo MA, Kegeles LS, Malone KM, Campbell CC, Sackeim HA, Mann JJ (2001) Decreased regional brain metabolism after ect. Am J Psychiatry 158:305–308
48. Pahapill PA, Lozano AM (2000) The pedunculopontine nucleus and Parkinson's disease. Brain 123(Pt 9):1767–1783
49. Pereira EA, Muthusamy KA, De Pennington N, Joint CA, Aziz TZ (2008) Deep brain stimulation of the pedunculopontine nucleus in Parkinson's disease. Preliminary experience at Oxford. Br J Neurosurg 22(Suppl 1):S41–S44
50. Rabins P, Appleby BS, Brandt J, DeLong MR, Dunn LB, Gabriels L, Greenberg BD, Haber SN, Holtzheimer PE 3rd, Mari Z, Mayberg HS, McCann E, Mink SP, Rasmussen S, Schlaepfer TE, Vawter DE, Vitek JL, Walkup J, Mathews DJ (2009) Scientific and ethical issues related to deep brain stimulation for disorders of mood, behavior, and thought. Arch Gen Psychiatry 66:931–937
51. Sankar T, Tierney TS, Hamani C (2012) Noval applications of deep brain stimulation. Surg Neurol Int 3:S26–S33
52. Seminowicz DA, Mayberg HS, McIntosh AR, Goldapple K, Kennedy S, Segal Z, Rafi-Tari S (2004) Limbic-frontal circuitry in major depression: a path modeling metanalysis. Neuroimage 22:409–418
53. Smith JR, Fountas KN, Murro AM, Park YD, Jenkins PD, Morrell M, Esteller R, Greene D (2010) Closed-loop stimulation in the control of focal epilepsy of insular origin. Stereotact Funct Neurosurg 88:281–287
54. Stefani A, Lozano AM, Peppe A, Stanzione P, Galati S, Tropepi D, Pierantozzi M, Brusa L, Scarnati E, Mazzone P (2007) Bilateral deep brain stimulation of the pedunculopontine and subthalamic nuclei in severe Parkinson's disease. Brain 130:1596–1607
55. Sun FT, Morrell MJ, Wharen RE Jr (2008) Responsive cortical stimulation for the treatment of epilepsy. Neurotherapeutics 5:68–74
56. Thevathasan W, Mazzone P, Jha A, Djamshidian A, Dileone M, Di Lazzaro V, Brown P (2010) Spinal cord stimulation failed to relieve akinesia or restore locomotion in Parkinson disease. Neurology 74:1325–1327
57. Tierney TS, Lozano AM (2013) Intervention options: functional neurosurgery. In: Morris ME, Iansek R (eds) Rehabilitation in movement disorders. Cambridge University Press, Cambridge
58. Tierney TS, Sankar T, Lozano AM (2011) Deep brain stimulation emerging indications. Prog Brain Res 194:83–95
59. Vitek JL, Jones R, Bakay R, Hersch S (2000) Pallidotomy for Huntington's disease. Ann Neurol 48:429
60. VNS Study Group (1995) A randomized controlled trial of chronic vagus nerve stimulation for treatment of medically intractable seizures. The Vagus Nerve Stimulation Study Group. Neurology 45:224–230
61. Weaver FM, Follett K, Stern M, Hur K, Harris C, Marks WJ Jr, Rothlind J, Sagher O, Reda D, Moy CS, Pahwa R, Burchiel K, Hogarth P, Lai EC, Duda JE, Holloway K, Samii A, Horn S, Bronstein J, Stoner G, Heemskerk J, Huang GD (2009) Bilateral deep brain stimulation vs best medical therapy for patients with advanced Parkinson disease: a randomized controlled trial. JAMA 301:63–73
62. Williams A, Gill S, Varma T, Jenkinson C, Quinn N, Mitchell R, Scott R, Ives N, Rick C, Daniels J, Patel S, Wheatley K (2010) Deep brain stimulation plus best medical therapy versus best medical therapy alone for advanced Parkinson's disease (PD SURG trial): a randomised, open-label trial. Lancet Neurol 9:581–591
63. World Health Organization (2001) Chapter 2: Burden of mental and behavioral disorders. In: The WHO report 2001: mental health, new understanding. New Hope. http://www.who.int/whr/2001/chapter2/en/Index3.html. Last Accessed on 28 Feb 2011
64. Zhang F, Gradinaru V, Adamantidis AR, Durand R, Airan RD, de Lecea L, Deisseroth K (2010) Optogenetic interrogation of neural circuits: technology for probing mammalian brain structures. Nat Protoc 5:439–456

Impact of Automated Hotspot Detection for ^{18}FET PET-Guided Stereotactic Biopsy

Thomas Reithmeier, Joacir Cordeiro, Michael Mix, Michael Trippel, Christoph Rottenburger, and Guido Nikkhah

Abstract *Objective*: The aim of this study was to explore the impact of automated hotspot detection on surgical planning of ^{18}FET PET-guided stereotactic serial biopsy.

Method: Imaging of ten patients with brain lesions detected by MRI and showing increased ^{18}FET uptake on PET who were retrospectively and randomly assigned to compose the study. Stereotactic biopsy plans (PET-guided and MR-guided) were performed by two neurosurgeons for each patient, independently and blinded. For PET-guided plans, biopsy target was achieved by means of an automated hotspot detection system. MR-guided plans targeted contrast enhancement areas or hyperintense areas in T2-weighted sequences. FET uptake ratio (UR) was determined in the biopsy trajectory across the lesion. Highest UR (HUR) from both planning techniques was compared.

Results: Each single HUR obtained through PET-guided technique was higher than correspondent values from MR-guided technique. Mean HUR of 2.41 (SE ± 0.23) for PET-guided plans and 1.85 (±0.16) for MR-guided plans were respectively obtained. This difference was statistically significant ($p = 0.002$).

Conclusion: The use of an automated hotspot detection system was able to provide higher FET HUR along stereotactic biopsy trajectories in comparison to those from MR-guided plans. The use of specially designed computational tools may refine surgical planning by improving biopsy targeting.

Keywords Stereotactic brain biopsy • Automated hot spot detection • FET-PET

Introduction

Stereotactic brain biopsy (SBB) has proven to be an efficient method to obtain histological specimens of newly diagnosed brain lesions with a very low complication rate. SBB is less invasive than open brain biopsy, and may be performed under local anaesthesia. Accurate histological diagnosis may avoid unnecessary brain resection of lesions that may mimic gliomas (e.g., brain lymphoma). There are some concerns about its diagnostic power in comparison to the primary resection of brain tumours, due to claimed sampling limitation of SBB. A few studies have addressed this issue by comparison of histological results received by stereotactic biopsy to subsequent open resection specimens, which found concordant rates between 51 and 79 % [2, 9, 12]. These studies were retrospective, and methodological drawbacks were observed.

Regardless of the technique chosen, brain biopsy is routinely performed using morphologic imaging guidance (e.g., MRI and/or CT scans). The role of PET imaging as a method to evaluate tumor metabolism is under investigation. PET is able to detect areas of increased tracer uptake (i.e., hotspots).

T. Reithmeier, MD (✉), J. Cordeiro, and M. Trippel, MD,
Division of Stereotactic and Functional Neurosurgery,
Department of Neurosurgery, Neurosurgical Clinic,
University Medical Center Freiburg,
Breisacher Straße 64, Freiburg D-79106, Germany
e-mail: thomas.reithmeier@uniklinik-freiburg.de

M. Mix and C. Rottenburger
Department of Nuclear Medicine, University Medical Center Freiburg, Freiburg, Germany

G. Nikkhah, MD, PhD
Division of Stereotactic and Functional Neurosurgery,
Department of General Neurosurgery, Neurosurgical Clinic,
University Medical Center Freiburg,
Breisacher Straße 64, Freiburg D-79106, Germany

Neurosurgical Clinic, University Hospital Erlangen,
Schwabachanlage 6, Erlangen D-91054, Germany
e-mail: guido.nikkhah@uk-erlangen.de

Thomas Reithmeier and Joacir Cordeiro contributed equally to the work described in this manuscript

DOI 10.1007/978-3-7091-1482-7_15,

Increased uptake ratio (UR) may be correlated to the presence of neoplasia and tumor grading. PET-guided biopsy (i.e., aimed at hotspots) might lead to the most metabolic active tumor areas. This might improve diagnosis accuracy, and reduce sampling errors due to non-optimal SBB targeting or missing of small malignant areas within large radiological uniform lesions.

A premise for the integration of PET into the surgical planning is a reliable coregistration of PET to stereotactic CCT or MR images. This is a demanding task, due to the different imaging profile of PET scans compared to MRI and CT scans. Moreover, due to relevant UR variation, searching for the area with highest UR may be imprecise and time-consuming if performed visually. New computational tools able to provide automatic PET imaging coregistration and three-dimensional automatic detection of areas harbouring highest UR could refine surgical planning. For this purpose, a PET planning module was developed coupled to the Inomed planning system. We here evaluated retrospectively UR profiles from MR-guided planning compared to those obtained through planning using the new automatic hotspot detection system.

Methods

The requirements for integration of metabolic information into the Inomed planning system for stereotactic planning procedures were defined by an interdisciplinary team of neurosurgeons, neuro-oncologists, nuclear physicians, nuclear physicists, and software developers. These included visualization of PET images, analysis of the standard uptake values along the trajectory according to the biopsy positions, automatic hot spot selection in a 2D and 3D environment, an automatic contouring of activity distribution within the tumor in relation to the hot spot, definition of reference areas for calculation of SUV (standard unified values) ratios, and a reporting system.

The development and integration of a PET module to the Inomed planning system was performed by a cooperative project between the University of Freiburg and Inomed, and included the following features:

Definition of Reference Areas

Uptake ratio (UR) is defined as the ratio between the mean SUV from the analyzed area and the mean SUV from an arbitrary reference area. For UR calculation, reference areas can be defined by the user with a freehand drawing tool. The reference area is characterized by mean, maximum, and minimum values as well as surface area in mm^2.

Visualization of PET Images

For standardized SUV visualization and interpretation a spectrum colorbar is used, where the lower and upper level are individually defined. This is especially important, as different tracers have different uptake patterns.

Analysis of SUV Along the Trajectory

Absolute SUV as well as UR along the planned trajectory in 1-mm steps are displayed in a separate window. The user can define the distance before and after the target point to be analyzed. Absolute SUV values are calculated on the basis of a circular area around the stereotactic coordinate on the trajectory. The radius of the circular area is defined by the user, and the absolute SUV value is calculated as the mean of all SUVs within this area. URs are also automatically calculated, and different reference areas can be selected by a drop-down menu.

2D and 3D Hot Spot Definition and Analysis

Usually the target point should be defined within the metabolic most active area of the tumor. Therefore, a software tool for automatic selection of the hot spot in a 2D and 3D environment was integrated. On axial PET slices, a circular area is defined for hot-spot detection that can be freely moved within this slice. The point with highest metabolic activity within this area is then automatically marked. When the 3D tool for hot-spot detection is activated, the circular area defined on the actual slice is transformed to a tube, and hot-spot detection is performed within this tube.

An additional feature is the possibility to analyze the metabolic distribution within the region of interest. This was realized by displaying isodose lines which delimitate an area with defined percentage of the maximum SUV. Up to three different isodose lines can be displayed within the region of interest, and the percentage values of all three isodose lines can be adjusted in one percentage step (Fig. 1d).

Patient Population

Ten patients without ring-enhancing lesions and a well-defined hot spot in ^{18}FET-PET examination who underwent stereotactic serial biopsy were retrospectively analyzed. The patient group was composed of eight male and two

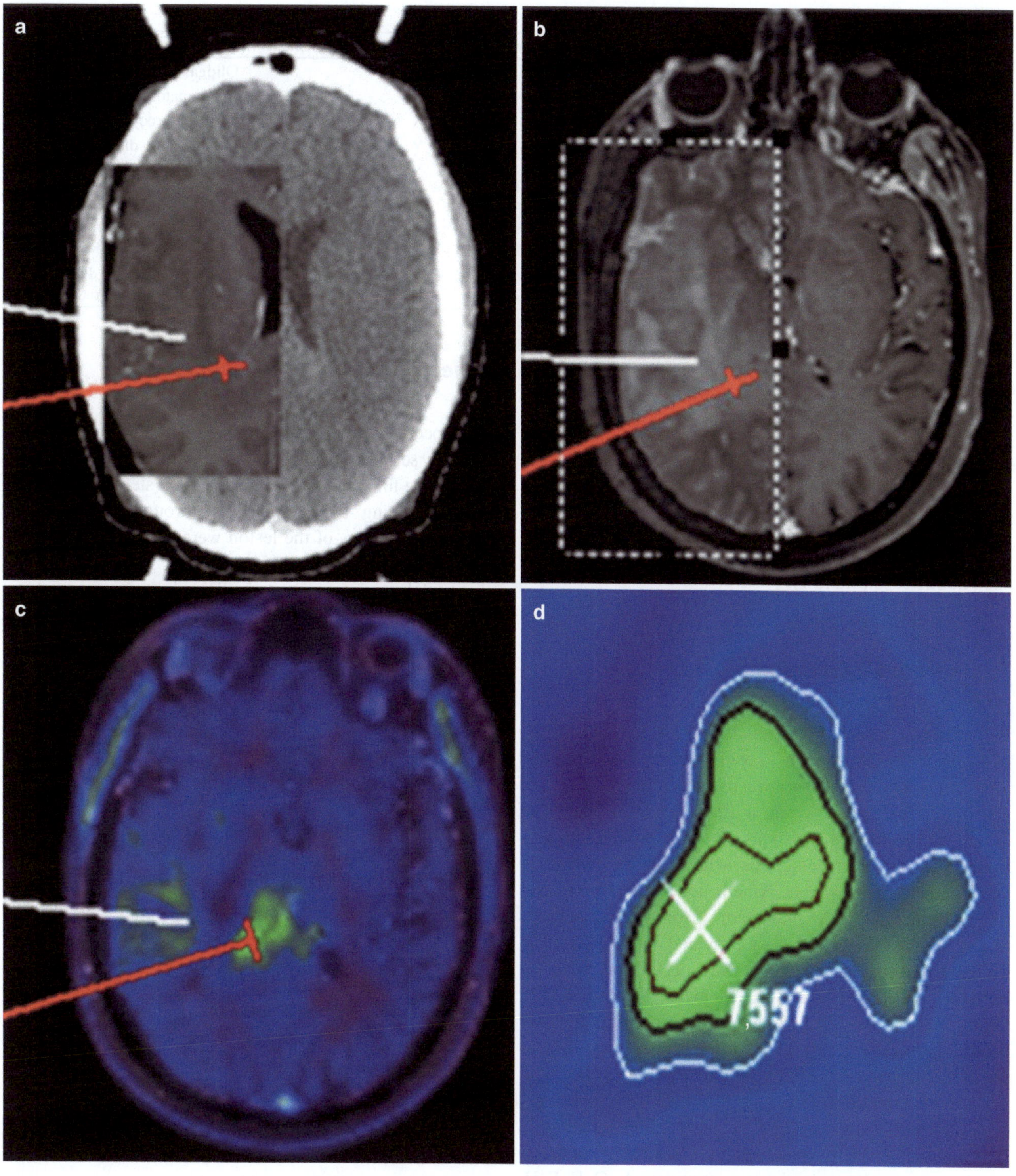

Fig. 1 *Red lines* illustrate PET -guided stereotactic approach, whereas *white lines* the MR-guided approach. **a** Automatic coregistration of frame-CT and T1-weighted MRI in which no tumoral contrast enhancement was observed on MRI. **b** Automatic coregistration of T1-weighted and T2-weighted MRI. Note the MR -guided approach targeting the hyperintense area in the T2-weighted sequence (*white line*). **c** Automatic coregistration of FET-PET-CT and T1-weighted MRI. Note the PET -guided approach (*red line*) targeting the tumor area with the highest FET uptake, which differed from the more superficial target aimed by the MR-guided approach. **d** Automatic drawn isolines at the areas corresponding to 70, 80, and 90 % (*red*, *black*, and *white* respectively) of maximum FET uptake 7,557 MBq/ml (*white cross*)

Table 1 Patients' characteristics

Patient	Age	Sex	Number of probes	Seizure	Focal deficit	Contrast enhancement	Histopathological diagnosis
A	27	M	11	Y	N	Y	Oliogastrocytoma grade II
B	32	F	17	N	Y	Y	Inflammatory disease
C	47	M	9	Y	N	N	Diffuse astrocytoma grade II
D	25	M	10	Y	Y	Y	Inflammatory disease
E	39	M	7	Y	N	N	Oligodendroglioma grade II
F	33	M	20	Y	N	N	Diffuse astrocytoma grade II
G	49	F	14	Y	Y	Y	Anaplastic astrocytoma grade III
H	38	M	16	N	Y	Y	Diffuse astrocytoma grade II
I	32	F	11	Y	N	Y	Oligodendroglioma grade II
J	56	M	15	Y	Y	N	Oligoastrocytoma grade III

female patients with mean age at surgery of 37.3 (±10.3) years. All patients presented symptomatic brain lesions. Seizures were present in eight patients and focal neurologic deficits in five. Histopathological evaluation revealed a diffuse astrocytoma grade II in three cases, an oligodendroglioma grade II in two cases, an inflammatory process in two cases, and an oligoastrocyomta grade II, oligoastrocytoma grade III, and an anaplastic astrocytoma grade III each in one case (Table 1).

Preoperative Evaluation

Pre-operative workup included 1.5 or 3.0 T MR imaging of 1-mm slices acquired in T1-weighted sagital sequences after intravenous administration of gadolinium. In cases of no-contrast enhanced lesion, a T2-weighted sequence of 1-mm sagital slices was also performed. Brain lesions presented contrast enhancement on MRI in six cases, and no enhancement in four cases. Nine lesions were supratentorial and one was in the brainstem. Prior to PET, patients fasted at least 6 h. FET was provided by EURO PET, Freiburg, Germany. Scanning was performed with an ECAT Exact 922 scanner (CTI/Siemens, Knoxville, TN, USA). A total of 250 MBq of FET were intravenously infused. Emission scans were performed in three-dimensional mode from 10 to 25 min after FET injection, with measured attenuation correction. PET data were iteratively reconstructed using OSEM reconstruction algorithm. Histological diagnosis obtained by stereotactic biopsies was low-grade glioma in six cases (patients A, C, E, F, H, and I), high-grade glioma in two cases (patients G and J), and non-specific inflammatory process in two cases (patients B and D).

Stereotactic planning was performed using the Inomed planning system (developed by Tatramed spol. s r.o. Bratislava, Slovak Republic, and Inomed, Emmendingen, Germany). Frame-CT was stereotactically transformed, and coregistered with preoperative MRI and FET-PET (Fig. 1a–c).

Trajectory Planning Procedure

Retrospectively, two neurosurgeons with experience in stereotactic serial biopsies performed surgical plans independently. The first neurosurgeon performed stereotactic biopsy plans, targeting the lesion only through MR. Contrast enhancement areas of the lesion were chosen as biopsy targets. In the cases where no contrast enhancement was observed, hyperintense areas in T2-weighted sequences corresponding to hypointense areas in T1-weighted sequences were targeted. The second neurosurgeon used the PET software module for target point definition, and target point coordinates were provided by automated detection of the area with highest FET uptake inside the hot spot (original PET trajectory). In cases where the target needed to be changed due to the presence of blood vessels, stereotactic coordinates were compared with those of the original PET-based trajectory (adjusted PET trajectory). Stereotactic coordinates obtained from MR-guided plans were compared with those from original and adjusted FET-PET-based trajectories. FET uptake was determined in the PET original and PET-adjusted biopsy trajectory by steps of 1 mm across the hot spot. The same procedure was performed after completion of the MR-guided plans in their biopsy trajectories. Highest (HUR) from both planning techniques were compared. Additionally, differences between the target point coordinates of PET-adjusted and MR-guided plans were calculated in all three axes (x, y, z).

Statistical Analysis

Statistical analysis was performed according to the advice of the Department of Statistics from the University of Freiburg. Results are presented in means ± standard error (SE). HUR obtained from ^{18}FET-PET and MR-guided techniques were analyzed using the sign test at a significance level of 95 % ($p<0.05$). For analysis, the SPSS software was used (SPSS Inc., Chicago, IL, USA).

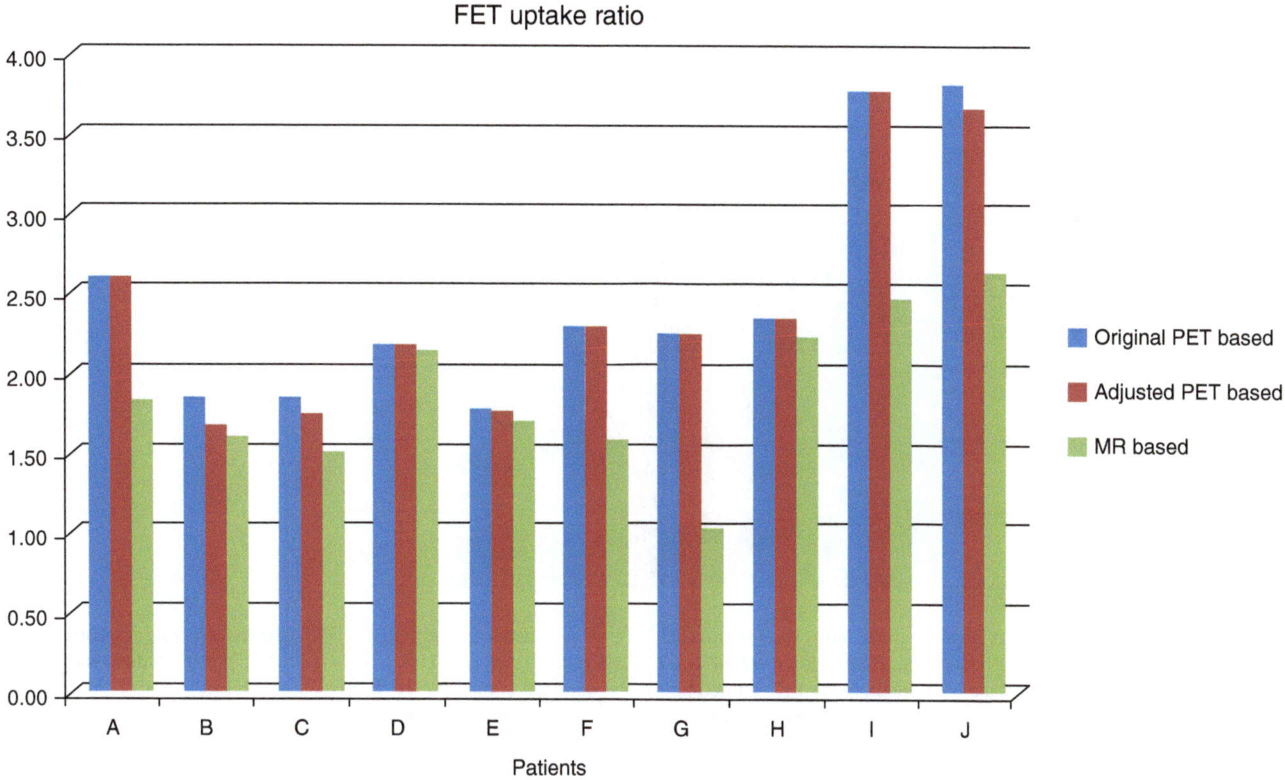

Fig. 2 FET uptake ratios were calculated dividing the FET uptake by a contralateral cortical reference. Highest FET uptake ratio (HUR) of original PET-guided stereotactic plan (*blue* columns) of each patient (A to J) was compared to HUR values obtained from PET-guided stereotactic plan adjusted to the presence of blood vessels (*red* columns) and to HUR values from MR-guided plans (*green* columns). Note that all values obtained through the MR-guided technique were inferior to both PET-guided techniques

Results

HUR from trajectories obtained from original PET-guided, adjusted PE-guided and MR-guided techniques were determined. Each single HUR obtained through the adjusted PET-guided technique was higher than the correspondent value from MR-guided technique (Fig. 2). Mean HUR values of 2.45 (±0.23), 2.41 (±0.23), and 1.85 (±0.16) respectively were obtained for the three techniques. Statistically significant higher HUR values were obtained from the adjusted PET-guided technique than from the MR-guided one ($p=0.002$). No significant statistical difference could be obtained comparing HUR with either PET-guided technique (Fig. 3).

In three cases, the area with highest metabolic activity could not be targeted due to the presence of blood vessels (patients B, C and J). Target variation between MR-guided and adjusted PET-guided techniques was, in stereotactic coordinates, horizontally 6.1 (±6.2) mm, vertically 6.8 (±6.0) mm, and in depth 7.0 (±7.2) mm. The highest and lowest variations were, respectively, horizontally 20.6 and 0.4 mm, vertically 16.5 and 0.3 mm and in depth 25.9 and 1.3 mm.

Discussion

Constant efforts are directed to improving diagnostic methods of a newly diagnosed intracranial lesion, by adding information about metabolic activity. Etiological diagnosis guided by conventional MRI has revealed high sensitivity, but a limited specificity for a neoplastic brain lesion around 68 %. It has been possible to increase the accuracy in distinguishing neoplastic from nonneoplastic tissue to 81 % through the use of MR imaging in conjunction with MR spectroscopy. With the addition of O-(2-[^{18}F]fluoroethyl)-L-tyrosine PET (FET-PET) to the conventional MRI, the specificity may be increased to 88 %. It has been possible to increase the accuracy in distinguishing neoplastic from nonneoplastic tissue to 97 % using MR imaging in conjunction with FET-PET and MR spectroscopy [5].

Increased FET uptake has been associated with reduction of *N*-acetylaspartate concentration, which represents loss of normal neurons [20]. FET is not incorporated into proteins, and shows high uptake by cerebral gliomas and squamous cell carcinomas due to increased transport phenomena [11]. In contrast to glucose derivatives, the uptake of amino acids in macrophages and other inflammatory cells is lower; thus,

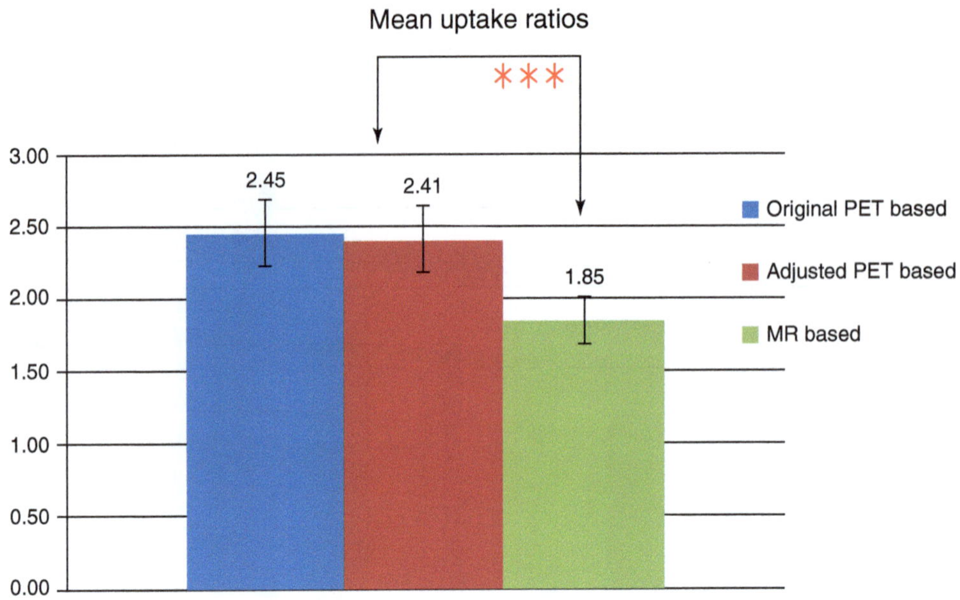

Fig. 3 In this figure, the mean of highest uptake ratio (HUR) from each stereotactic planning technique is depicted. *Blue* column refers to the original PET-guided technique, the *red* column to the PET-guided plan adjusted to the presence of blood vessels, and the *green* column to the MR-guided technique. Statistically significantly higher HUR values were obtained from the adjusted PET-guided technique compared to the MR-guided one ($p=0.002$). No significant statistical difference could be obtained comparing HUR from both PET-guided techniques. Data displayed in means ± standard error

amino acid tracers appear to be more specific than 2-[^{18}F]fluoro-2-deoxy-D-glucose (FDG) for tumor imaging [4]. Studies comparing FET and MET uptake in brain tumors brought comparable results [19, 21]. Due to the short physical half-life of the ^{11}C-label, ^{11}C-Methionine PET (MET-PET) remains restricted to a few centers with a cyclotron on site, differently from FET which is suitable for routine clinical practice [8].

FET-PET belongs to the current workup of patients harbouring newly diagnosed brain lesions in many centres, despite variable rates of sensitivity and specificity. FET-PET findings from 14 patients were considered positive in five glioma patients, but also in three out of nine patients with nonneoplastic lesions, including two patients with brain abscesses and one with a demyelinating lesion [6]. Cerebrovascular disease represents another important differential diagnosis in brain lesions suspected to be gliomas, and increased uptake of amino acids such as FET or MET has been described in ischemic brain lesions [10, 13, 18]. FET-PET dynamic techniques are highlighted in comparison to standard techniques. In a series of 45 glioma patients, individual time course analysis of FET uptake was able to diagnose and differentiate low-grade from high-grade recurrent astrocytomas with a sensitivity and specificity of 92 % [16].

The use of PET is not limited to diagnostic purposes, it may also refine surgical technique, improve follow-up and facilitate tumor delimitation for radiotherapy planning [5, 7, 14, 17]. The use of a pre-operative FET-PET helps to identify regions with abnormally increased metabolic activity, which may differ from MRI contrast enhancement areas. This was the case of four patients in our series where two biopsy targets were needed due to MRI and FET-PET discordance. In two out of these four patients, histological findings obtained from the FET-PET active area revealed tumor upgrading, which wouldn't have been diagnosed if sampling was limited to the contrast-enhanced areas [3]. Patients with infratentorial brain lesions may also profit from pre-operative metabolic imaging. Twenty children with newly diagnosed intrinsic infiltrative brainstem lesions underwent PET-guided stereotactic biopsy. The use of PET-guided trajectories could provide a histological diagnosis or higher tumor grading in comparison to MRI -guided planning [15].

By adding FET-PET imaging to guide a stereotactic biopsy, surgical planning and target point definition may be relevantly influenced, which may have a significant impact on the histological result. An illustrative example is the case of one patient from our study. This patient harbored a brain tumor, which presented no contrast enhancement, and therefore T2-weighted sequences were used to perform MR -guided stereotactic biopsy planning. The MR-guided target differed from the one obtained by the PET-guided plan, which was more profound. This correlates to the past medical history of this patient, in which she first underwent open brain biopsy which was nondiagnostic. Afterwards, she underwent FET-PET-guided stereotactic biopsy. According to preoperative FET-PET imaging, the target point was defined in the posterior corpus callosum, and histological analysis revealed the presence of anaplastic astrocytoma (Fig. 1).

Further data with regard to correlation of FET uptake ratio and tumor grading are needed to evaluate sensitivity and specificity of FET-PET imaging in the primary diagnosis of brain lesions and in follow-up. A prospective study of 11 glioblastoma patients showed a FET UR of 3.16 (±0.75) which was statistically significantly different from a theoretical value of 2. In this series, a mirrored brain area and normal gray matter were used as reference [1]. A larger series of 54 patients submitted to dynamic PET revealed FET UR of 2.16 (±0.98) for low-grade and 3.29 (±1.06) for high-grade gliomas. In this study, contralateral cortex was used as reference [17]. Studies comparing FET and MET UR in malignant gliomas and brain metastasis brought comparable results around 2.7 (±0.8). FET uptake in normal gray matter and white matter was 1.1 (±0.2) and 0.8 (±0.2) respectively [21]. We believe that a more precise correlation between FET UR and histological characteristics (e.g., cellular density, presence of necrosis and proliferation index), as well as a systematic analysis of different references, could improve non-invasive diagnostic methods. Due to the lack of optimal sensitivity and specificity, the "gold standard" in the workup of a new diagnosed brain lesion remains the histological analysis.

Conclusion

The use of an automated hot-spot detection system was able to provide higher FET HUR along stereotactic biopsy trajectories than those from MR-guided plans. The use of specially designed computational tools as used in the present study may refine surgical planning by improving biopsy targeting of undefined lesions of the central nervous system.

Acknowledgments This work was financially supported by a grant from Inomed, Emmendingen, Germany. Authors would like to thank Dr. Graf from the Department of Statistics of the University of Freiburg for the support in the statistical analysis.

Conflict of Interest Cordeiro JG was financially supported by Inomed to perform systematic evaluation of computational tools developed for the neurosurgical practice. We confirm that we have read the Journal's position on issues involved in ethical publication, and affirm that this report is consistent with those guidelines.

References

1. Benouaich-Amiel A, Lubrano V, Tafani M, Uro-coste E, Gantet P, Sol JC et al (2010) Evaluation of O-(2-[^{18}F]-fluoroethyl)-L-tyrosine in the diagnosis of glioblastoma. Arch Neurol 67(3):370–372
2. Candrasoma PT, Smith MM, Apuzzo ML et al (1989) Stereotactic biopsy in the diagnosis of brain masses: comparison of results from biopsy and resected surgical specimen. Neurosurgery 24:160–165
3. Cordeiro JG, Rottenburger C, Pinsker M, Trippel M, Weber W, Nikkhah G, Reithmeier T (2010) Value of ^{18}F-FET PET in comparison to stereotactic serial biopsy to evaluate the follow up of brain gliomas. Presented in the 19th congress of the European Society Stereotaxic and Functional Neurosurgery, Athens
4. Del Sole A, Falini A, Ravasi L, Ottobrini L, De Marchis D, Bombardieri E et al (2001) Anatomical and biochemical investigation of primary brain tumours. Eur J Nucl Med 28:1851–1872
5. Floeth FW, Pauleit D, Wittsack H et al (2005) Multimodal metabolic imaging of cerebral gliomas: positron emission tomography with [^{18}F]fluoroethyl-L-tyrosine and magnetic resonance spectroscopy. J Neurosurg 102(2):318–327
6. Floeth FW, Pauleit D, Sabel M et al (2006) ^{18}F-FET PET differentiation of ring-enhancing brain lesions. J Nucl Med 47(5):776–782
7. Grosu AL, Weber WA, Franz M et al (2005) Reirradiation of recurrent high-grade gliomas using amino acid PET (SPECT)/CT/MRI image fusion to determine gross tumor volume for stereotactic fractionated radiotherapy. Int J Radiat Oncol Biol Phys 63(2): 511–519
8. Hamacher K, Coenen HH (2002) Efficient routine production of the ^{18}Flabelled amino acid O-(2-[^{18}F]fluoroethyl)-L-tyrosine. Appl Radiat Isot 57:853–856
9. Jackson RJ, Fuller GN, Abi-Said D et al (2001) Limitations of stereotactic biopsy in the initial management of gliomas. Neuro Oncol 3:193–200
10. Jacobs A (1995) Amino acid uptake in ischemically compromised brain tissue. Stroke 26:1859–1866
11. Langen K, Hamacher K, Weckesser M et al (2006) O-(2-[^{18}F]fluoroethyl)-L-tyrosine: uptake mechanisms and clinical applications. Nucl Med Biol 33(3):287–294
12. Mc Girt MJ, Villavicencio AT, Ketan RB, Friedman AH (2003) MRI-guided stereotactic biopsy in the diagnosis of glioma: comparison of biopsy and surgical resection specimen. Surg Neurol 59:277–282
13. Nakagawa M, Kuwabara Y, Sasaki M, Koga H, Chen T, Kaneko O et al (2002) 11C-Methionine uptake in cerebrovascular disease: a comparison with ^{18}F-FDG PET and 99mTc-HMPAO SPECT. Ann Nucl Med 16:207–211
14. Pauleit D, Stoffels G, Bachofner A et al (2009) Comparison of (18)F-FET and (18)F-FDG PET in brain tumors. Nucl Med Biol 36(7):779–787
15. Pirotte BJM, Lubansu A, Massager N et al (2007) Results of positron emission tomography guidance and reassessment of the utility of and indications for stereotactic biopsy in children with infiltrative brainstem tumors. J Neurosurg 107(5 Suppl):392–399
16. Pöpperl G, Kreth FW, Herms J et al (2006) Analysis of ^{18}F-FET PET for grading of recurrent gliomas: is evaluation of uptake kinetics superior to standard methods? J Nucl Med 47(3):393–403
17. Pöpperl G, Kreth FW, Mehrkens JH et al (2007) FET PET for the evaluation of untreated gliomas: correlation of FET uptake and uptake kinetics with tumour grading. Eur J Nucl Med Mol Imaging 34(12):1933–1942
18. Rottenburger C, Doostkam S, Prinz M, Meckel S, Nikkhah G, Meyer P, Reithmeier T (2010) Interesting image. Amino acid PET tracer accumulation in cortical ischemia: an interesting case. Clin Nucl Med 35(11):907–908
19. Rottenburger C, Hentschel M, Kelly T, Trippel M, Brink I, Reithmeier T, Meyer PT, Nikkhah G (2011) Comparison of C-11 methionine and C-11 choline for PET imaging of brain metastases: a prospective pilot study. Clin Nucl Med 36(8):639–642
20. Stadlbauer A, Prante O, Nimsky C et al (2008) Metabolic imaging of cerebral gliomas: spatial correlation of changes in O-(2-^{18}F-fluoroethyl)-L-tyrosine PET and proton magnetic resonance spectroscopic imaging. J Nucl Med 49(5):721–729
21. Weber WA, Wester HJ, Grosu AL et al (2000) O-(2-[^{18}F]fluoroethyl)-L-tyrosine and L-[methyl-11C] methionine uptake in brain tumours: initial results of a comparative study. Eur J Nucl Med 27(5): 542–549

Interstitial Radiosurgery with Iodine-125 Seeds in the Treatment of Brain Metastases, Glial Tumours and Benign Intracranial Lesions

Michael Trippel, Thomas Reithmeier, and Guido Nikkhah

Abstract In a retrospective single-centre study, we analysed data of 1,378 patients (55 % male, 45 % female) who underwent interstitial radiotherapy with 1,596 implanted Iodine-125 seeds in the Department of Stereotactic and Functional Neurosurgery in Freiburg from January 1990 to December 2011. The medical prerequisites and physical parameters of the treatment with Iodine-125 seeds are given. The method used in Freiburg relying on temporary Iodine-125 seed implants is described in detail and analysed. The survival rates and the peri-operative risk are evaluated. We conclude that interstitial radiosurgery with Iodine-125 seeds is a safe and useful tool, offering a wide range of treatment options for benign and also malignant intracranial lesions, especially if they are small, deep-seated, in eloquent areas, or not suitable for micro-surgery.

Keywords Brachytherapy • Iridium-192 • Iodine-125 • Seeds • Interstitial radiotherapy • Stereotactic biopsy • Glioma • Low-grade glioma • Brain tumours • Metastases • Hamartoma • Child • Adults • Survival • Adverse events

M. Trippel, MD (✉) and T. Reithmeier, MD
Division of Stereotactic and Functional Neurosurgery,
Department of Neurosurgery, Neurosurgical Clinic,
University Medical Center Freiburg, Breisacher Straße 64,
Freiburg D-79106, Germany
e-mail: michael.trippel@uniklinik-freiburg.de

G. Nikkhah, MD, PhD
Division of Stereotactic and Functional Neurosurgery,
Department of General Neurosurgery, Neurosurgical Clinic,
University Medical Center Freiburg,
Breisacher Straße 64, Freiburg D-79106, Germany

Neurosurgical Clinic, University Hospital Erlangen,
Schwabachanlage 6, Erlangen D-91054, Germany
e-mail: guido.nikkhah@uk-erlangen.de

Introduction

Interstitial radiosurgery (IRS) with iodine seeds, a form of brachytherapy (brachy derived from the Greek meaning "short") is an internal radiotherapy where a radiation source is placed inside or nearby a radiosensitive lesion for treatment. Brachytherapy has a long and well-established tradition in the Department of Stereotactic and Functional Neurosurgery in Freiburg [2, 3, 5–15]. In a retrospective study, we analysed data of all the patients that underwent brachytherapy treatment with Iodine-125 Seeds in Freiburg from 1990 to 2011.

In earlier years, permanent implants of Iridium-192 made from thin flexible wires (5) that could be cut to any length were implanted by a stereotactic procedure. Iridium-192 has a half-life of 73.83 days, a mean energy of 380 keV, and half value layer of ~65 mm in tissue. Iodine-125 seeds used nowadays are sized 4.5 × 0.8 mm with 59.43 days half-life, delivering much lower photon energy in the range of 27.4–35.5 keV. These seeds contain Iodine-125 adsorbed onto a radio-opaque silver rod hermetically encapsulated in a welded titanium capsule. Typically available apparent activities range from 1 to 25 mCi. Due to their favourable physical properties and high attenuation (half value layer ~17 mm) in tissue, these seeds present a sharp dose decline and are therefore well-suited for the treatment of small (10–30 mm) intracranial lesions, also nearby eloquent and radiosensitive structures. The lower photon energy and thereby high natural absorption in tissue has the additional advantage that surrounding persons get a radiation exposure far below 1 mSv, which generally can avoid shielding and isolation of patients.

Methods

In a retrospective single centre study, we analysed data of all 1,378 patients (55 % male, 45 % female) who underwent interstitial radiotherapy with 1,596 implanted Iodine-125 seeds in

G. Nikkhah and M. Pinsker (eds.), *Stereotactic and Functional Neurosurgery*, Acta Neurochirurgica Supplement, Vol. 117,
DOI 10.1007/978-3-7091-1482-7_16,

the Department of Stereotactic and Functional Neurosurgery in Freiburg from January 1990 to December 2011.

For analysis of the influence of patients' age, they were assigned to the following four groups: Children (age 1–17, mean 9.46 ± 4.54 years, $n=297$, 21.5 %), adults (age 18–65, mean 40.15 ± 12.88 years, $n=934$, 67.8 %), seniors (age 66–90, 72.23 ± 5.16 years, $n=147$, 10.7 %) and a group of all patients (age 1–90, mean 36.96 ± 22.55 years, $n=1,378$, 100 %).

Treatment Procedure with Iodine-125 Seeds

In our centre patients are admitted the day before surgery. A frameless, non-reformatted magnetic resonance tomography (MRT) (MP-Rage, T1 weighted, sagittal, 1 mm, post gadolinium and T2-Space, sagittal, 1 mm, Avanto, Siemens, Erlangen/Germany) and if applicable a positron emission tomography (PET) are done and transferred to the planning workstation (STP3 Workstation, Stryker Leibinger, Düsseldorf/Germany). Next, the stereotactic base ring is fixed under local anaesthesia and a stereotactic computed tomography (CT) (Siemens Somatom Plus, Erlangen/Germany) post iodine contrast (Solutrast 100) is acquired with fiducials (Inomed, Emmendingen/Germany) fixed to the base ring. A stereotactic transformation and three-dimensional reconstruction are calculated; either image fusion of CT-scan, T1- and T2-weighted MRI is done using anatomical landmarks co-registration, or fully automatic image fusion (Precisis Plus Workstation, Inomed, Emmendingen) is performed. The segmentation of the external contour of the head, of the lesion, and of all radiosensitive organs at risk (e.g., eyes, chiasm, optic nerves and tracts, brainstem, pituitary stalk) is done; the dose at the surface of the lesion and the dose limitations for the organs of risk are prescribed. In most patients, a dose of 60 Gy is applied to the surface of the lesion. Then planning is simulated using one or more Iodine seeds. The seeds delivering the prescribed dose in about 30 days are selected. The actual implantation time and stereotactic target coordinates are optimized first automatically then manually using isodose diagrams and 3D-modeling, respecting eloquent areas and blood vessels for the implantation tracts. The selected Iodine-125 seeds are taken from the radiation protection vault. The calculated radiation activity is controlled by measuring the seeds. The seed is heat-shrunk into the end of a Teflon catheter and autoclaved in a radiation-shielded container.

The stereotactic serial biopsy is done using a small skin incision, a 6 mm burr-hole typically following the tract of the seed catheter. The planned target position of the seed is retained by fluoroscopy in two planes using a stereotactic probe. The centre of the autoclaved seed within the catheter is implanted exactly at the target position under fluoroscopy control. The seed catheter is fixed in the burr hole using either fibrin foam or bone cement with a radio-opaque haemoclip. The skin is closed in two layers by a suture. For high precision, positioning of the seed can be controlled by an intra-operative native CT scan and image fusion with the treatment plan. The radiation emission is measured and documented at distances of 0, 20, and 100 cm to the body's surface according to legal rules. If applicable, the patient is instructed to avoid long-lasting and close contacts (<1 m) with pregnant women and children. Rules for surrounding persons are given to ensure a radiation exposure far below 1 mSv during total implantation time, in compliance with legislation and regulations. As a general rule, an isolation of the implanted patients is not necessary. The patients are dismissed the second day after surgery. If no contraindications apply, we use short-term antibiosis (e.g., Cefuroxim, 1.5 g, intravenous) during seed implantation. A possible reactive brain oedema can be treated using oral administration of low-dose steroids (e. g., dexamethasone).

Investigations have been done in the treatment of malignant brain tumours (glioma and sarcoma) in dogs which favour temporary seed implants [7]. Therefore, at the end of the implantation period, possibly after a MRI control, the seed with the catheter and the haemoclip are removed by a small skin incision under local anaesthesia taking only a few minutes. After explantation of the seed, macrophage activity will increase, inducing further shrinking and degradation of the tumour necrosis over the following months. This has to be taken into account in the interpretation of subsequent PET, CT, and MRI imaging to avoid the false positive diagnosis of tumour progression.

Localization of the lesions

The implanted lesions were localized in the frontal (336), temporal (257), parietal (167), occipital (41) lobes, the basal ganglia (129), thalamus (32), hypothalamus (57), diencephalon (106), pons (26), lower brainstem (8), midbrain (86), pineal region (10), cerebellum (25), and ventricle (32). Most of the treatments took place on the left side (650, 47.2 %) compared on the right side (611, 44.3 %), the midline (36, 2.6 %) and bilaterally (13, 0.9 %).

Histopathological Diagnosis

The implantation of the iodine seed was preceded by a stereotactic serial biopsy in 1,111 (80.6 %) patients in the same procedure. Due to conclusive preoperative neuroradiological findings, stereotactic biopsies were less frequent in patients with craniopharyngioma (33.3 %), tumours of the pineal region (57.1 %), and in patients with pharmacoresistant gelastic epilepsy with typically located hypothalamic hamartoma (53.3 %). The mean number of biopsy samples taken was 7.31 ± 3.14 for the whole group, ranging from 5.55 ± 3.20 for hypothalamic hamartoma to 9.4 ± 5.46 for glioblastoma.

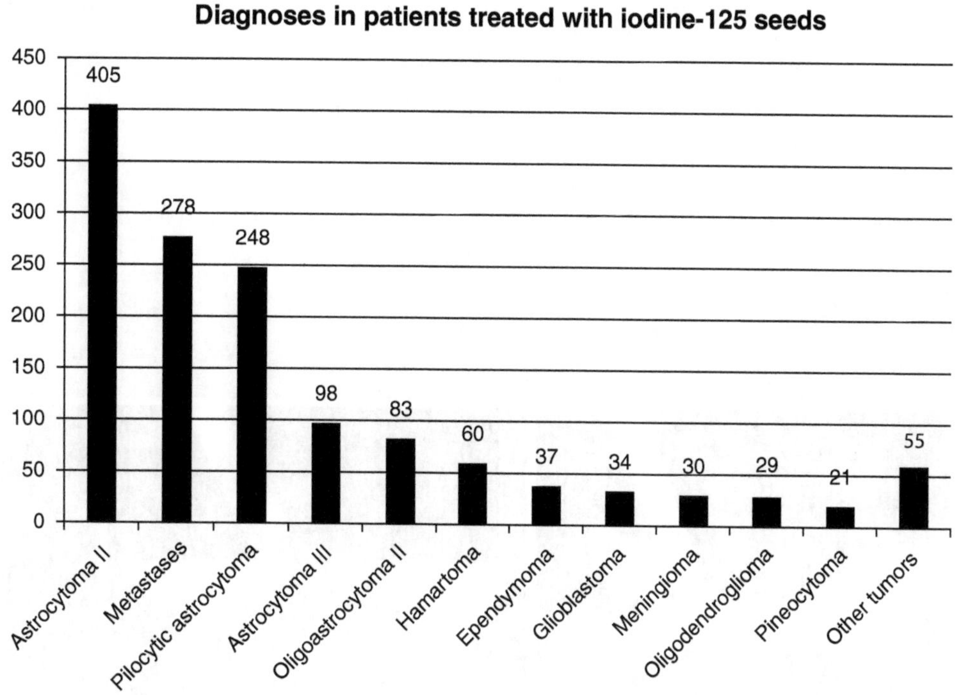

Fig. 1 Frequency of diagnoses in patients with intracranial lesions treated with Iodine-125 seeds

The most frequent histo-pathological findings were fibrillary astrocytoma (405; 29.3 %), metastasis (278; 20.1 %), pilocytic astrocytoma (248; 18.0 %), anaplastic astrocytoma WHO III (98; 7.1 %), oligoastrocytoma WHO II (83; 6.1 %), hamartoma (60; 4.3 %), ependymoma (37; 2.7 %), glioblastoma (34; 2.5 %), meningioma (30; 2.2 %), oligodendroglioma (29; 2.1 %), and tumours of the pineal gland (21; 1.5 %) (Fig. 1).

In the children group (n=297), there was a predominance of pilocytic astrocytoma (162; 54.6 %), fibrillary astrocytoma (73; 24.6 %), hypothalamic hamartoma (20; 6.73 %), and oligoastrocytoma (10; 3.4 %). Korinthenberg et al. analysed a subgroup of 94 children (mean age 9.0 years) with deep-seated low-grade glioma that underwent implantation of temporary seeds with 53.6 (6.8–171.0) months follow-up [1, 2, 4, 16].

In the group of adults (n=934), the most frequent diagnoses were fibrillary astrocytoma (326; 34.9 %), metastases (178; 19.1 %), pilocytic astrocytoma (86; 9.2 %), astrocytoma WHO II (83; 8.9 %), oligoastrocytoma WHO II (70; 7.5 %), hypothalamic hamartoma (40; 4.3 %), ependymoma (28; 3.0 %), and oligodendroglioma (23; 2.5 %).

In the senior group (n=147), the most frequent lesions were metastases (100; 68 %), malignant (15; 10.2 %) and low-grade glioma (14; 9.5 %), and meningioma (11; 7.5 %).

Physical Treatment Parameters

The physical parameters for the implanted seeds were analysed. Their activity ranged from 0.7 to 68.9 mCi; the mean was 12.17 ± 7.08 mCi, the median 11.5 mCi. There are lesions that deviate significantly from the mean activity. Much lower activity was used for gangliocytoma (n=8, 6.73 ± 3.52 mCi) and for hypothalamic hamartoma (n=60, 3.6 ± 1.73 mCi), due to the smaller volume of the lesion. A higher activity was selected for anaplastic astrocytoma (16.25 ± 9.52 mCi) and in glioblastoma (14.16 ± 9.89 mCi), due to the larger size of the lesions and higher malignancy.

The mean energy dose rate used was 9.63 ± 2.21 cGy/h. A slightly lower dose rate was used for gangliocytoma (8.15 ± 0.73c Gy/h) and craniopharyngioma (8.5 ± 2.12 cGy/h). The mean lay time of the seeds was 29.6 ± 14.63 days, for meningioma 34.24 ± 12.85 days, and for oligodendroglioma 34.34 days. The mean prescribed dose at the surface of the tumour was 60.48 ± 4.41 Gy, the median dose 60 Gy, the maximum dose 100 Gy. Doses in the range from 60 to 100 Gy were only used in 27 (1.95 %) patients with malignant glioma.

The mean number of seeds per treatment was 1.16 ± 0.4 for all patients, in glioblastoma 1.37 ± 0.77, in anaplastic astrocytoma 1.26 ± 0.54, and in fibrillary astrocytoma 1.25 ± 0.46. The maximum number of seeds per treatment was five for glioblastoma, and four seeds for pilocytic, fibrillary, and anaplastic astrocytoma.

Repetitive Treatments

The mean number of treatments per patient with iodine seeds was 1.15 ± 0.42 for the whole group. More recurrent treatments were necessary for hypothalamic hamartoma (n=60: 1.57 ± 0.60, range 1–3), for ependymoma (n=37: 1.27 ± 0.52, range 1–3) and for gangliocytoma (n=8: 1.5 ± 0.58, range 1–2).

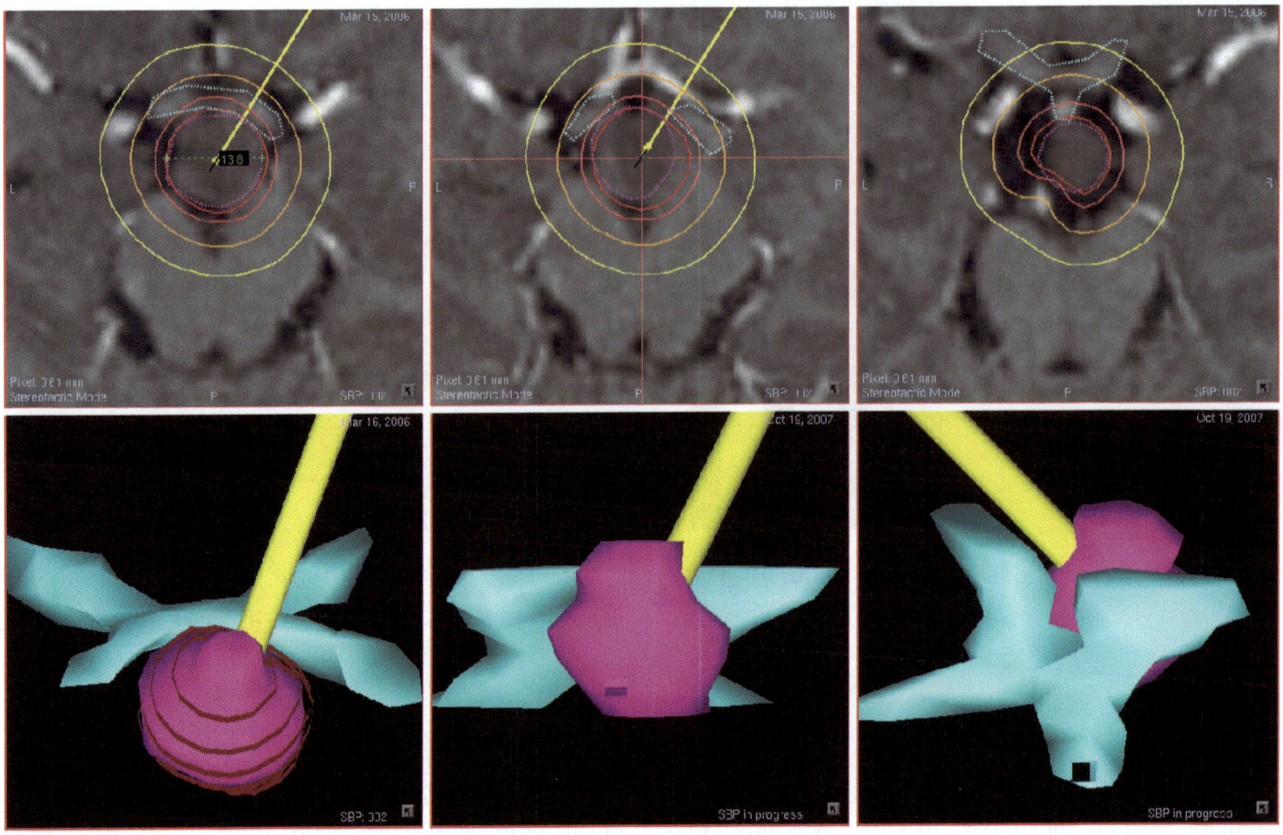

Fig. 2 The treatment plan for a stereotactic biopsy with subsequent implantation of an Iodine-125 seed in a patient with a hypothalamic hamartoma suffering from long-term pharmacoresistant gelastic epilepsy is shown. The *upper line* gives three horizontal MRI views; in the *lower line*, three-dimensional reconstructions are displayed. The chiasm, the optic nerves, the optic tracts, the pituitary stalk, the hypothalamic hamartoma, the stereotactic approach, and the isodose lines are visualized. The 60 Gy isodose line is visible on the surface of the tumour

Size of the Lesions

The mean diameter of all lesions was 21.34 ± 6.32 mm; larger mean diameters were found for anaplastic astrocytoma (24.04 mm), craniopharyngioma (26.54 mm), and meningioma (24.06 mm), and smaller for hypothalamic hamartoma (11.96 mm) and gangliocytoma (17.5 mm).

The mean volume of the lesions was 6.41 ± 5.18 ml. Larger volumes were found for craniopharyngioma (10.21 ± 4.51 ml) and anaplastic astrocytoma (8.85 ± 6.51 ml), and smaller for hypothalamic hamartoma (1.07 ± 0.85 ml) and for gangliocytoma (3.23 ± 2.08 ml). The maximum volume treated was 24.4 ml in a metastasis not suitable for open micro-surgery.

Costs and Resources

The patients underwent implantation of their seed in 77.5 % of cases under local anaesthesia, and in 22.5 % under general anaesthesia. For all patients with frequent seizures and for most children, we preferred general anaesthesia, making general anaesthesia more frequent in hypothalamic hamartoma (63 %) and pilocytic astrocytoma (62 %).

The mean time for a serial stereotactic biopsy including waiting for the intra-operative histo-pathological diagnosis, with subsequent implantation of the iodine seeds including the intra-operative computed tomography control, was 62 ± 36 min. Without biopsy and histo-pathological examination, the time was reduced to 28 ± 8 min. This makes stereotactic biopsy with subsequent seed implantation a cost- and time-efficient procedure.

Selected Clinical Series

Treatment of Hypothalamic Hamartoma

Since 1998, patients with hypothalamic hamartoma suffering from pharmacoresistant seizures were treated by the implantation of iodine seeds in Freiburg [17–20]. We compared interstitial radiotherapy to LINAC-radiosurgery and micro-surgery. The patients treated with seeds had a good outcome, with very low procedure-related morbidity rate, with good hypothalamic and neuro-cognitive function, and without any fatalities. In some patients when treatment planning for LINAC radiosurgery had to be discontinued due to local over-dosage at the chiasm and the optical tracts, treatment with iodine seeds was still feasible based on the higher homogeneity and sharp dose decline at the surface of the hamartoma.

Figure 2 shows a treatment plan for the implantation of an Iodine-125 seed with stereotactic biopsy in a patient suffering from long-term pharmacoresistant gelastic epilepsy. The 60 Gy isodose line is visible on the surface of the tumour.

Brainstem Lesions

In the whole group, 120 patients had lesions of the brainstem which were treated with iodine seeds, thereof 86 in the midbrain, 26 in the pons, and eight in the lower brainstem; 73 patients presented with glioma, thereof 37 with pilocytic astrocytoma, 21 with metastases, and 26 with other tumours; 25 were children (20.8 %).

Survival

Survival data of 1,098 patients is available. In the whole group of 1,378 patients, 65 died within the first 100 days, 12 within a month, and three within a week following the treatment with an iodine seed. Sixty out of these 65 patients suffered from extra-cranial metastases; five died from their malignant glioma.

This could suggest the exclusion from intra-cranial treatment with iodine seeds of patients with poor life expectancy due to an extended extra-cranial metastatic spread.

The survival rate at 5 and 10 years in a subgroup of 94 children with deep-seated glioma treated by temporary seed implants investigated by Korinthenberg et al. was 97 and 92 % [1]. These results are quite comparable to those of other centres applying brachytherapy, with a survival rate of 93 and 82 % given in [16].

Procedure-Related Adverse Events

During implantation of the seed under local anaesthesia, five patients presented focal seizures that were successfully treated with intravenous application of diazepam not requiring the abortion of the procedure. One patient showed a minor reaction following the application of iodine contrast, one had a procedure-related epidural haematoma, 12 showed minor intracerebral haematoma, thereof one requiring subsequent open surgery, and two other patients presented a postoperative hemiparesis. One patient died due to bleeding in a metastasis of a malignant melanoma following the explantation of a seed.

The risk of a possible infection of the seed implant can easily be minimized by autoclaving the seed within the catheter, and by a peri-operative short term intravenous antibiosis.

Discussion

Interstitial radiosurgery with Iodine-125 seeds is a safe, minimally invasive, well-tolerated, cost- and time-efficient neurosurgical procedure with a very low rate of adverse events, low temporary and permanent morbidity and fatalities. Except for children, 92.5 % of the patients underwent seed implantation under local anaesthesia, thereby saving human and technical resources. If no histo-pathological diagnosis is available, an additional stereotactic biopsy can easily facilitate the diagnosis at low risk and minimal additional effort. Lesions, especially in highly eloquent areas like the brainstem, thalamus, basal ganglia, hypothalamus, near the chiasm and optic tracts, which often are not suitable for micro-surgical resections are still easily accessible to a stereotactic biopsy and subsequent interstitial radiotherapy with iodine seeds. For children under the age of 10 with small intracranial lesions, treatment with Iodine-125 seeds offers a well-tolerated possibility for a circumscribed high-dose local radiotherapy, avoiding by its specific sharp dose decline many of the negative side-effects of external radiotherapy to the developing juvenile brain. For the same reason, brachytherapy offers, in a subgroup of patients in case of malignant tumour recurrence, options for salvage therapy when the dose limitations of external fractionated radiotherapy are already reached.

Conclusion

Interstitial radiosurgery with Iodine-125 seeds is a safe and useful tool in the hands of specially trained stereotactic neurosurgeons in particular centres. It offers a wide range of treatment options for benign and also malignant intracranial lesions, especially if they are small, deep-seated and difficult to approach for open micro-surgery, or when biological limitations or age restrictions apply for the use of external fractionated radiotherapy.

Acknowledgements I want to thank my teacher Professor Dr. C. B. Ostertag for giving us deep insights in the significance, practice, and handling of iodine seeds. We thank Professor M. Schumacher and his distinguished team from the Department of Neuroradiology, University Medical Centre Freiburg for their cooperation, and for providing us with excellent MRI imaging. Vera Gumpp from the Tumorzentrum

Ludwig Heilmeyer, Comprehensive Cancer Center Freiburg (CCCF), University Medical Centre Freiburg supplied us with precise and controlled survival data. We thank Ms. Manuela Fellmann for her excellent work in the preparation of the International Congress on the occasion of the 60th anniversary of Stereotactic Neurosurgery in Freiburg, and for the handling of our manuscripts for this supplement.

References

1. Korinthenberg R, Neuburger D, Trippel M, Ostertag C, Nikkhah G (2011) Long-term results of brachytherapy with temporary iodine-125 seeds in children with low-grade gliomas. Int J Radiat Oncol Biol Phys 79:1131–1138
2. Kreth FW, Faist M, Warnke PC, Rossner R, Volk B, Ostertag CB (1995) Interstitial radiosurgery of low-grade gliomas. J Neurosurg 82:418–429
3. Kreth FW, Faist M, Rossner R, Birg W, Volk B, Ostertag CB (1997) The risk of interstitial radiotherapy of low-grade gliomas. Radiother Oncol 43:253–260
4. Moringlane JR, Graf N, Ostertag CB (1987) Stereotaxic diagnosis of brain tumours in childhood as a principle for therapy planning. Klin Padiatr 199:260–268
5. Mundinger F, Ostertag CB, Birg W, Weigel K (1980) Stereotactic treatment of brain lesions. Biopsy, interstitial radiotherapy (iridium-192 and iodine-125) and drainage procedures. Appl Neurophysiol 43: 198–204
6. Ostertag CB, Weigel K, Mundinger F (1981) Computer tomographic course controls after brain tumour radiotherapy. Strahlentherapie Sonderb 76:119–124
7. Ostertag CB, Warnke P, Kleihues P, Bigner DD (1984) Iodine-125 interstitial irradiation of virally induced dog brain tumours. Neurol Res 6:176–180
8. Ostertag CB (1987) Interstitial stereotactic radiotherapy of brain tumours. Wien Klin Wochenschr 99:380–384
9. Ostertag CB (1989) Stereotactic interstitial radiotherapy for brain tumours. J Neurosurg Sci 33:83–89
10. Ostertag CB, Kreth FW (1992) Iodine-125 interstitial irradiation for cerebral gliomas. Acta Neurochir (Wien) 119:53–61
11. Ostertag CB (1993) Central nervous system injury from implanted isotopes. Recent Results Cancer Res 130:209–217
12. Ostertag CB (1993) Brachytherapy-interstitial implant radiosurgery. Acta Neurochir Suppl (Wien) 58:79–84
13. Ostertag CB (1994) Stereotaxic radiosurgery. Nervenarzt 65: 660–669
14. Ostertag CB (1994) Interstitial implant radiosurgery of brain tumours: radiobiology, indications, and results. Recent Results Cancer Res 135:105–116
15. Ostertag CB, Kreth FW (1995) Interstitial iodine-125 radiosurgery for cerebral metastases. Br J Neurosurg 9:593–603
16. Ruge MI, Simon T, Suchorska B, Lehrke R, Hamisch C, Koerber F, Maarouf M, Treuer H, Berthold F, Sturm V, Voges J (2011) Stereotactic brachytherapy with iodine-125 seeds for the treatment of inoperable low-grade gliomas in children: long-term outcome. J Clin Oncol 29:4151–4159
17. Schulze-Bonhage A, Homberg V, Trippel M, Keimer R, Elger CE, Warnke PC, Ostertag C (2004) Interstitial radiosurgery in the treatment of gelastic epilepsy due to hypothalamic hamartomas. Neurology 62:644–647
18. Schulze-Bonhage A, Quiske A, Homberg V, Trippel M, Wagner K, Frings L, Bast T, Huppertz HJ, Warnke C, Ostertag C (2004) Effect of interstitial stereotactic radiosurgery on behavior and subjective handicap of epilepsy in patients with gelastic epilepsy. Epilepsy Behav 5:94–101
19. Schulze-Bonhage A, Trippel M, Wagner K, Bast T, Deimling FV, Ebner A, Elger C, Mayer T, Keimer R, Steinhoff BJ, Spreer J, Fauser S, Ostertag C (2008) Outcome and predictors of interstitial radiosurgery in the treatment of gelastic epilepsy. Neurology 71:277–282
20. Schulze-Bonhage A, Dennig D, Wagner K, Cordeiro JG, Carius A, Fauser S, Trippel M (2010) Seizure control resulting from intrahippocampal depth electrode insertion. J Neurol Neurosurg Psychiatry 81:352–353

Author Index

DOI 10.1007/978-3-7091-1482-7, © Springer-Verlag Wien 2013

R

S

W

Y

Subject Index

MIX
Papier aus verantwortungsvollen Quellen
Paper from responsible sources
FSC® C105338

If you have any concerns about our products,
you can contact us on
ProductSafety@springernature.com

In case Publisher is established outside the EU,
the EU authorized representative is:
Springer Nature Customer Service Center GmbH
Europaplatz 3, 69115 Heidelberg, Germany

Printed by Libri Plureos GmbH
in Hamburg, Germany